Dear Reader,

Since I wrote this book almost one year ago, much has progressed in our quest to prove that low level light therapy (LLLT), also known as photobiomodulation, helps Alzheimer's patients improve cognition, and appears to slow or stop and stabilize degeneration.

Additionally, the use of neurofeedback, specifically LORETA Z Score neurofeedback based on a quantitative electroencephalogram (QEEG) can double the effect of light therapy in improving cognition. Each work well on their own, but together each doubles the performance of the other.

It appears to some scientists that the cause of Alzheimer's is an energy shortfall, and that near infrared light therapy, which goes through the cranium, and increases the production of ATP, the fuel of the cell, in the mitochondria. This empowers the cells and the brain to many vital things that older, senescent cells may not have the energy to do. And, as was discovered in Europe, when cells do not have this minimal electrical state to stay health, they seem to get sick, and die. We surmise that the build-up of amyloid plaque may be a downstream result of this energy shortfall. Scientists are looking at this, but government and industry is still focused on the potential for drugs and implanted devices based on the failed amyloid plaque model.

To induce change and awareness we have to conduct a study of 100 humans. Medicine is stuck in old paradigms, and unless you have evidence you are not believed. Evidence based medicine is not a good indicator when promising breakthroughs are not funded because the funder does not believe in them. Catch-22. The innovations are sacrificed for the belief systems that are sacred.

As it turns out, the technologies that help with Alzheimer's and TBI are already cleared by the FDA as safe, but not for Alzheimer's, or TBI. We need support from patient advocates to get this study funded. The breakthroughs in technology were funded by the US Army, and conducted by the Veteran's Administration, in studying traumatic brain injury, working with scientists at Harvard who have led the study of photobiomodulation. They have been stalled for years, not getting to soldiers or patients.

The most significant finding to date is this ten minute video. You will see how neurons get very excited and busy when a near infrared light is put on the head. The QEEG records the activity.

Watch this video and listen to the scientist speaking to understand how and why light therapy works. www.vielight.com/neurofeedback.

I and many others have decided that this particular light device, the Vielight Neuro, either Alpha or Gamma, works the best of any, as it includes a number of important design advantages having to do with the position of the light, the pulsing, and frequency and the power. In this book I show a variety of devices ranging from $200 to $5,000, and all can help induce the effect shown, safely, that will help those with Alzheimer's and TBI, but science is not ready to agree, nor to fund studies. I am now convinced that the Vielight device is the best bet for improving getting energy into the brain, which appears to help Alzheimer's more than any drug to date. But is not funded by the industry that controls healthcare in America. It is being studied and used in other countries.

The Vielight Neuro ranges in cost from $1400 to $1750. A 10% discount is available to my readers if you put my name, Weiner, in as the discount code.

Hence I am updating this book with several new pieces of data.

The first study in humans showing the positive effects of light therapy on nine humans with Alzheimer's was just released, and can be read here:

https://app.box.com/s/ccm2cl52fk6u6yaz9j8ij6nj51zq128p

Here is information on the study clinicians are planning for both those with Traumatic Brain Injury (TBI) and Alzheimer's: https://app.box.com/s/smwjytsfbl0tsm9rzy9pxwpj7jwqzihq Write to us at studyTBIandAD@gmail.com to get on the list for more information. The plan is to have the study approved and underway in April, 2017.

It takes money to do this. We estimate that a one-year study of 100 patients with TBI or Alzheimer's may cost $2 million, or $20,000 each. We need to raise capital and hope that foundations and others will help us fund this. 501c3 tax deductible gifts can be made to one of several foundations supporting this effort, such as the Quietmind Foundation at www.quietmindfdn.org. Measureable, positive results occur in only 60 days.

The second addition are some charts created by a former Boston Scientific Director of R&D showing why certain frequencies of light are important, and why they get through the cranium.

The third is a slide show about an experimental study of the light and neurofeedback in 100 or more patients that is being organized and will start in Florida, Philadelphia, Texas, California, New York, and Washington state, this year, under the auspices of an Internal Review Board. Studies can be undertaken in any city where there are twenty or more patients that will enroll, and a patient advocate group to fund the study, which can be undertaken by visiting a clinic twice weekly. I do not have all the information as yet, but you can write to studyTBIandAD@gmail.com and get on the list to be informed as to study details.

Both the light therapy and neurofeedback are on the market, and affordable. So is an FDA approved device for treating depression with transcranial magnetic energy, and the ultrasound machines that are used to image the babies in the womb, all are safe, and help with Alzheimer's. However, science and medicine are so overregulated and stuck in their ways, that this opportunity to help millions of people suffering from Alzheimer's, more than suffer from cancer and diabetes combined, has lied fallow for years, while a small contingent of dedicated scientists and clinicians has pressed on.

While I believe the NIH rightfully should undertake the cost of this study, they are caught up in the complicated politics that has them doing the bidding of Big Pharma, and consciously ignoring this evidence. And device companies want invasive implants, not a low cost solution as light and neurofeedback. They are working on adapting deep brain magnetic stimulation (DBMS) technology used for Parkinson's to provide Alzheimer's patients with the energy needed to improve their health. But it is not necessary to implant the electrode deep in the brain, when shining light on the skull works. They prefer the risk of a major operation that is unnecessary, but highly profitable, and with a protected channel of neurosurgeons.

We are getting this information out to the public so this unnecessary, expensive and dangerous procedure is not foisted on the population when low cost, safe, non-invasive technology will do the job. Americans are particularly abused by a system of big corporations profiteering I very complicated medical technologies. However, this simple, yet glaring example of malfeasance in industry and government may break the monopoly. Here is evidence that can help the reader see through the scam.

This is essential, as healthcare is not a business doing life saving healing by any means. This technology represents an existential threat to Big Pharma and the makers of pacemakers and heart pumps, who charge a great deal of money to offer obsolete and outdated technology rather than compete and offer the most efficacious, and life saving innovations in their arsenal. They have no obligation to develop or ship the best. Their board members and shareholders want growth in profit and market share. No one asks if they can make more efficacious devices. They can. That is one reason why the price is so high. It does not need to be. Capitalism works best with competition, and healthcare is not competitive and has no sense or urgency, or will to win. Science is also too slow and complacent. The funding does not encourage innovation, but relies on drugs that are complex, expensive, and can be dangerous.

Many things stand in the way of innovation, but none as inexcusable as the fact that light therapy can stave off the Alzheimer's pandemic. Once you arrange to get a light and use it, you should try and find a trained practitioner of LORETA Z score neurofeedback, using QEEG of the brain compared to a normalized database of individuals. The neurofeedback resets the brain and tunes the brainwaves towards optimization. That is why this therapy also helps with drug addiction, ADHD, depression, epilepsy and autism (search for neurofeedback and any of these and see for yourself).

Best of luck to the reader in sorting through the inefficiency of healthcare and medicine to find something that works, but is not profitable enough for a non-competitive, usurious, profitable industry bigger than can be efficient, or controlled. By educating the public about the facts and the failings of medicine in the face of non-competitive giants, perhaps change will ensue.

That is the hope of this little book.

Here is a paper from a leading Harvard scientist on the potential for photobiomodulation:
https://app.box.com/files/0/f/17394711176/1/f_132630011639

In fact, light provides the most efficient regenerative medicine. See this:
https://app.box.com/s/inomdpnkho89wbw02fhzy97fvk0zci4m

To summarize what is now known and not believed by the bureaucracy of medicine:

OPPORTUNITY TO TREAT ALZHEIMER'S IN HUMANS

1. Study in press has shown that photobiomodulation (PBM), aka Low Level Light Therapy (LLLT) improves cognition in Alzheimer's patients (see attached).

2. Studies have shown that transcranial magnetic stimulation (TMS), approved by the FDA for treating depression, has a 6-point increase in the COG scale from only 6 weeks of therapy, on Alzheimer's patients. (A 2 Tesla device out of Israel has been approved for fast track at the FDA. It will require transporting patients to the clinic for therapy).

3. Studies at the University of Arizona have shown that transcranial ultrasound (TUS), using low power imaging devices, has positive therapeutic effects on Alzheimer's patients.

4. Studies have shown cognitive improvements in patients using non-regulated neurofeedback therapy.

5. Use of neurofeedback with light therapy has shown that each double the output of the other. (Light therapy appears to slow and stabilize degeneration.)

6. DOD funded studies conducted by the VA and Harvard have shown that PBM and neurofeedback each, individually, improve Traumatic Brain Injury (TBI) in patients.

7. Studies in Israel show that light therapy improves neuronal growth in nerve pads, dendrites, and synapses.

8. The ability of light energy to cause cells to increase their uptake can affect both their efficacy and their reduction of potential overdose. (Covered this in our pending IP.)

9. This opportunity represents a next generation potential in medicine comparable to the pacemaker, the stent or the medical robots from Intuitive.

10. There are certain activation points within the energy spectrum that can generate incremental cellular activity through ATP, and up and down regulation of genes, having an impact on cell biology that can be directed and controlled. We call this our digital pharmacopeia.

11. Due to the concentration by the medical industry in invasive procedures (pharmaceutical, surgical and implantable), this opportunity was missed.

12. Our intentions are to collaborate with partners licensing out to several segments, internationally, favoring entrepreneurs with capabilities and access to the giants of industry, with their overhead and fear of engagement.

LUMINEU, INC.

Lumineu is a newly formed company which has acquired the patent portfolio from NooThera, the venture which created the IP under the guidance of Irv Rappaport, former Chief Patent Counsel at Medtronic. The patents are all under PCT international coverage.

They have filed on the opportunity for combinatorial use of these frequencies and energies to be shown to produce better outcomes than the single purpose studies cited above. Many energies and methodologies are included, including up and down regulation of genes, and the uptake of pharmaceuticals, nutraceuticals, vitamins, et al as the result of the light energy on cell activity.

While some technologies, such as near-infrared light, have been both patented and shown in the literature to have certain effects, prior to Lumineu's 2015 patent filings. the combination of light plus neurofeedback has not been reported in the literature, nor has the very effective combinations of ultrasound and light therapy, transcranial magnetic stimulation, in combination, including with neurofeedback. Patent protection is essential in getting the private sector to offer a solution through regulated medicine.

Studies have shown that the light therapy also induces increased ATP as well as inducing increased growth of mesenchymal stem cells.

Studies have been done in mice for Alzheimer's and are successfully growing kidneys in animals and is regenerating heart tissue in human stroke patients in human in Israel, using light induced healing.

Lumineu is organizing a privately funded study of neurofeedback with PBM, for both TBI and Alzheimer's disease, to end the debates and show what actually works.

CONTACT

studyTBIandAD@gmail.com

REFERENCE

Robert Crowley, former BSCI Director R&D, now CEO of Soundwave Research on the Lumineu SAB:

To explain where the opportunity emerges that causes multiple energies to safely improve biological function, we offer this overview:

1. human body light absorption curves for 3 tissue components

2. solar terrestrial irradiance.

3. no chart needed. observed therapeutic effects of lightwaves to heal/repair/regenerate.

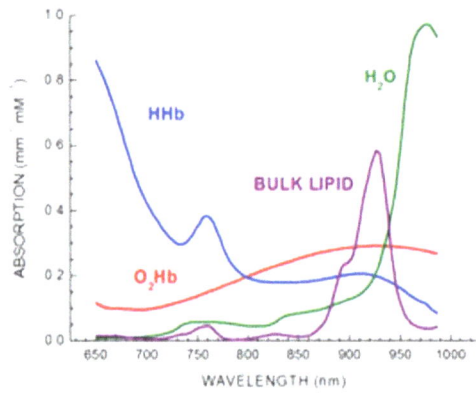

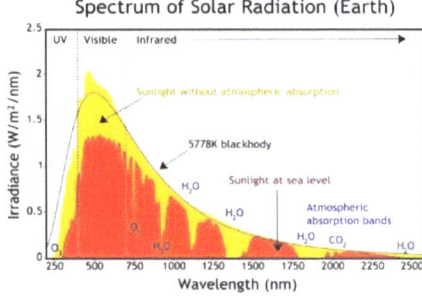

Info on Lumineu, Company PPT, SAB, patents, et al

The Light.

How Low Level Light therapy (LLLT) healed my Traumatic Brain Injury (TBI), and the struggle to deliver this remedy to those with Alzheimer's Disease.

The technology studied by the US Army and Harvard can stop and stabilize degeneration from **Alzheimer's,** and neurofeedback brings back memory.

This is the story of how we are fighting to get it into the clinic.

Table of contents

INTRODUCTION

Low level light therapy (LLLT, aka photobiomodulation) helps with Traumatic Brain Injury (TBI), as shown in years of study by the US Department of Defense (DOD), led by the US Army. There is growing evidence that it may also be the breakthrough for stopping the pandemic of Alzheimer's.

Alzheimer's is in many ways an affliction worse than cancer, for the individual with the degenerative disease, and their loved ones. Because, with cancer, you at least have your memories. Alzheimer's also affects more human beings, which most people do not realize (see chart on page 39).

Scientists are often the most wary. Thinking the energy can't possibly penetrate the skull (it can, and is well reported in the literature), can't possibly interfere with the degenerative process, but it does.

By supplying needed energy to neurons, at the right frequency as known by those working in the field of low level light therapy (LLLT), an increase in the growth of nerve pads, dendrites, and synapses in neurons, in both animals *and* humans, has been measured (see S. Rochkind at U. Tel-Aviv).

Studies in humans with Alzheimer's show statistically significant improvement, but the reaction of caregivers is closer to astonishment.

A great deal is being learned about neuroscience, biophysics, and brain plasticity, so that those who do not look at the exciting early indicators are slowing the path of progress, as is too often the case with innovation, particularly in medicine. But this technology is not received well by those in charge of science and medicine, for age old reasons.

Light is just one form of wave that can penetrate the body and affect biology. PEMF, TUS, TMS, and millimeter-waves all have been well reported in the scientific literature has having beneficial, therapeutic and curative effects.

They all have something in common, with what DARPA, the innovation arm of American defense, calls "directed energy." It healed my TBI injury, restored my memory, and there are strong indicators that low level light therapy (LLLT), LED and/or laser, plus neurofeedback, can stop Alzheimer's. This is especially promising with new PET imaging, before first memory loss. We can begin to slow, stop and stabilize degeneration before the debilitating losses occur.

My situation is more as an entrepreneur who has worked in fast pace innovation for many years, then switched to medical devices. My path was seemingly inadvertent, starting with a meeting with a scientist in Vienna in 2014 who provided the first clue that it is energy that is the missing supplement in the degeneration of the brain, that appears to cause amyloid plaque as the outcome of the deficiency, and not the reverse.

Unlike many people who suffer from memory loss from Traumatic Brain Injury (TBI) and Alzheimer's, I was lucky to be helping a team of scientists who had developed a therapy for stopping degeneration and improving cognition using energy where it was working in early human clinical trials.

"How did you hurt your head?" the technician giving me a demonstration of the equipment asked me.

"I didn't hurt my head," I explained, "I am just here for a demonstration, to understand how the equipment works."

"No, you hurt your head. Look at the screen, at the upper left frontal lobe." There was a clear discoloration, but it meant nothing to me.

"You appear to have suffered a traumatic brain injury,' he noted and then asked, "did you know that you are four to eight times more likely to develop early stage dementia as a result of a traumatic brain injury?"

"No! I did not know," I replied, "but the only head injury I ever had was when I was 15, and woke up in the hospital with a concussion, having slipped on the ice, and hit my head. But, it was in the back of the head," I explained.

"Coups contra coups," he said, using the term about the brain when it is impacted on one side and bruised on the opposite side.

This turned out to a very fortuitous interaction, because, six months later, while on a conference call, I could not recall how to push the necessary buttons to bring on another person on my iPhone. And my ability to remember names, and synonyms, was disappearing before my mind. It is a frightening experience, comes on rapidly, and then, you forget more, and more.

I fortunately recalled the things that I had learned on a due diligence trip to Vienna, Austria, a few years earlier, that had led to my working with scientists in Philadelphia and New York City, affiliated with NYU.

What I had learned about therapies working in laboratories in labs that were treating depression, tinnitus, ADHD, PTSD, TBI, epilepsy, autism and Alzheimer's, let me know where to get the non-regulated but effective neurofeedback therapy, and how to buy a device that provided the safe directed energy, in the form of infrared, and near-infrared (NIR).

The device used low level light therapy (LLLT), in the form of a 120 LED red light at a 660 nanometer wavelength. I learned later that 810-830 might have been better. These all work by impacting electron transfer and ion flow at the cellular level. Increasing mitochondria output of ATP (the fuel of the cell), and other changes.

Richard Satava, MD, a former DARPA program manager, first suggested to me that these therapies were actually using light frequency, not just the usual conception of light itself, to up and down regulate genes. Increasing ATP, VEGF, NO, and other vital precursors to healing.

Using the combined technology invented by a scientist in Philadelphia, I was able to recover my faulty memory, completely, in only six weeks of twice weekly therapy, not covered by insurance, but not very expensive.

I added weekly brain scans and other tests of cognitive progress/decline, which showed that my abnormal brainwaves returned to normal, my memory recovered and has stabilized. It has now been over a year and 6 months as of this writing in 2016.

I have been very fortunate to have been involved with clinicians working with a solution working in human studies. We discovered several other working solutions shown in studies in humans to work, and slow or stop the decline of Traumatic Brain Injury (TBI), with much evidence, and Alzheimer's with some.

However, industry and government are not working to get these to market. This is a sad situation for the many soldiers and football players afflicted with the disease. It is much worse for the 5 million Americans, and 40 million worldwide, with Alzheimer's.

The technology has been tried with Alzheimer's patients, and works. But that is not enough. Acceptable studies take time, and cash. Evidence based medicine sounds very scientific but not when bias derides a solution that seems to work in most people it has been tried with, in allowable studies done by FDA approved IRB's (Institutional Review Boards).

What sounded questionable actually stops and stabilizes degeneration, safely, and without contraindication. Non-invasively. However, publication grade studies require funding. And science and publication are not free.

The pharmaceutical and medical device industries thrive by working with invasive, or minimally-invasive solutions. Non-invasive? Sounds less profitable. It's not, but that is another first impression we have to contend with. And the business of medicine is summed up in several quick assessments. Does it work?

Is it proprietary, that is, are there patents? And, companies ask, do they have a channel to get to the neurologists, surgeons or psychiatrists, who can prescribe this? Is there a code (ICD-10), to get paid for the healing? And, do you have overwhelming evidence, taking the risk out, so we can make money, with certainty?

Healing is the least important aspect in this mercenary equation. Companies are rated on P&L, not outcomes (which is how to change the industry, btw).

Getting technology to the clinic is the work of those with swagger, who block the path of those who care about outcomes. Hippocrates is a socialist to these people. Do no harm limits channels and competitive advantage.

Why and how this discovery, now over ten years old since the first human double blind, placebo controlled studies were conducted, with statistically significant results, and ignored, may surprise you, as they did me.

Let me first show you what works, and then explain why a therapy clearly working for TBI is not on the market. The Alzheimer's solution also works, but bumps up against a scientific theory not proven (that amyloid plaque is the cause), that has deterred testing the one solution that works in humans most times it has been tried, and without the problems often caused by drugs, or surgery.

I will explain why it is not on the market, and may never be. Unless we, as consumers, get educated and upset and force medicine to look at what data and evidence there is. We have to change the rules of engagement in medicine, from a primary focus on what makes money, and is within the scientific comfort zone of the status quo, to one of what best heals, and then make money getting it to the clinic.

This is my introduction, and reason for writing this book. I will first explain the four technologies working in clinics for TBI, and why indications make them very promising.

I will tell you about meetings with government agencies, industry giants, large non-profit Foundations, and others.

All lacking both a sense of urgency and a belief in anything other then pharmaceuticals to possibly have a chance.

Norm Doidge, MD's's book on How the Brain Heals Itself (2007), and the Brain that Changes Itself (2016) detail with great human poignancy the revolution in neuroscience underway around the nation and the globe.

Through the publication of this book I hope that the promising technologies and the brave scientists, engineers and clinicians discovering this solution that stops Alzheimer's, will be recognized as such.

I am anticipating that more people will learn of this technology and demand it, and that the healthcare industry may change, develop a sense of urgency, and remember the teachings of Hippocrates, to do no harm.

Wherever possible I have provided links to useful information on the Internet.

Even if there is a great deal of money to be made in avoiding that ancient credo. There is much to be made from innovation and disruption in a classic industry.

That is the potential I hope this book will facilitate.

THE SOLUTION TO ALZHEIMER'S AND TBI THAT NOBODY WANTED

To fully understand the opportunity, and the inefficiency, we have to first look at traumatic brain injury (TBI), where there is great evidence of an effective therapy, and an amazing lack to action to get it to the millions in need. Particularly our soldiers and football players.

Then, when we look at Alzheimer's, we encounter another problem that makes things more complicated, amyloid plaque, tau and fibroidal tangles. This had been the focus of most research and funding. It is a false indicator. It would be like trying to cure scurvy in modern times without looking at the evidence of vitamin C.

It is here where assumptive, often arrogant belief in the process avoids the evidence, and bias occludes logic. Exactly what scientists wish to avoid, or so many say, while avoiding the evidence at hand and becoming devil's advocates, versus patient outcome advocates.

Getting evidence takes money, and the money goes to where the non-evidentiary, and often assumptive, belief systems, lead us. In science, it is not a quest for outcomes, it is a quest for funding, that uses up much of the efforts of scientists and institutions. "Go where the money is," is one of the worst quiet teachings of young Ph.D.'s and post docs.

Turning On Lights to Stop Neurodegeneration: The Potential of Near Infrared Light Therapy in Alzheimer's and Parkinson's Disease

Daniel M. Johnstone [1], Cécile Moro [2], Jonathan Stone [1], Alim-Louis Benabid [2] and John Mitrofanis [2*]

Department of Physiology, University of Sydney, Sydney, NSW, Australia, [2] University Grenoble Alpes, CEA, LETI, CLINATEC, MINATEC Campus, Grenoble, France, [3] Department of Anatomy, University of Sydney, Sydney, NSW, Australia

I have been in such innovation battles for over forty years, and have achieved some big wins, both scientifically, and financially, in areas of technology where my only qualification to participate was as a driven entrepreneur.

My involvement with medical devices began when I teamed up with Wilson Greatbatch*, the inventor of the first successful implantable pacemaker, licensed to a small, undercapitalized company in the 1960's, That small company, Medtronic, grew to prominence, and is now one of the largest medical device companies in the world.

In 1999 Wilson and I started working to solve the intractable contraindication of pacemakers to compatibility with MRI imaging. This seemingly obscure limitation of patients with pacemakers getting MRI's caused some people, such as those with colon cancer or a brain tumor, to be denied using MRI to identify the best, and safest means, to stage margins and detect successful excisions. It was a problem that bothered Wilson, as the pacemaker inventor, and Raymond Damadian, the inventor of MRI imaging.

Years later my company convinced Medtronic to purchase the technology, and the 74 pending and issued patents we had generated.

Four years later, in 2011, Medtronic announced the first in a series of MRI conditionally safe devices. Pacemakers, defibrillators and neurostimulators.

Wilson died three months after Medtronic launched the world's first conditionally safe pacemaker compatible with MRI, in 2011, at 92. Wilson had three times changed medicine. With no degrees in medicine he revolutionized it, several times, with his ingenuity and persistence. First the implantable pacemaker, then the long lasting lithium iodine battery for medical devices, doubling pacemaker useful life, and then the achievement of MRI safe pacemakers and neurostimulators. Here is a great story about the great man's life: http://www.electrohealing.com/about/wilson-greatbatch-memorial/greatbatch-articles/

I wish to illuminate a cultural problem that is manifesting itself as a chasm between scientists and the industry they serve.

30,000 Americans die each month from the failure of science and industry to look outside the box. These may seem like harsh words, but, there is a solution, and it is not properly reflected in the refereed literature, because proper, publishable studies take time and money. There was one, which has not published, but is being prepared and should publish soon. It tested 11 human patients and produced significant results. Other scientists derided having only 11 humans in a 30 day study, rather than seeing the value of a desperately needed clue.

They want the certainty of data, but would not fund evidence to fully vet the promise of innovation in the lab.

To explain where the solution to Alzheimer's and TBI can lead, I wish to tell you about another exciting and recent discovery about the use of low level light therapy (LLLT), or photobiomodulation, PBM, using light at specific nano-wave-length frequencies, shined on human bones in live people.

Light causes an activation of stem cells (mesenchymal), to grow faster in red bone marrow. These stem cells know where to go, and what do do. Using this same technology, ATP, the fuel of the cell, gives the body the energy to rebuild damaged heart tissue, working today, in humans!

Here is a publication about that seemingly unrelated study:
Lasers stimulate stem cells and reduce heart scarring after heart attack, study suggests https://www.sciencedaily.com/releases/2011/08/110811083820.htm

Additional Paper on stopping Alzheimer's, Parkinson's et al:
http://journal.frontiersin.org/article/10.3389/fnins.2015.00500/full

THAT ALSO WORKS FOR STOPPING THE DEGENERATION OF ALZHEIMER'S.

Infrared light at certain frequencies between 800 and 1200 have been shown in clinical trials to slow or stop TBI, and one paper is about to publish with statistically significant results in Alzheimer's.

Amazingly, the light sources do not have to be implanted. Light can be shined directly onto the cranium, will pass through the skull (the hair and scalp are actually more resistant than the skull), and cause a marked change in degeneration and stabilize the brain's condition if used regularly (every other day).

NEUROFEEDBACK

The addition of neurofeedback, specifically the type called LORETA Z score neurofeedback, will tune the brainwaves back into optimal performance, restoring some memory and personality at virtually any stage of decline.

Both of these technologies are readily available from neurotherapists (see bci-a.org or isnr.org)

However, it be claimed that this can help people survive, unless a specific device goes through the very expensive FDA approval process.

Light technologies are not on the market, other than for sports medicine, chiropractors, or veterinarians.

A search of low level laser therapy (LLLT) across the literature will show that the technology has miraculous effects on gum tissue, when used by dentists, and can even can regrow teeth by causing the release of stem cells, improves athletes' knees and horses' knees, but does not hardly exist in orthopedic practices for human knees.

It is the same across most of medicine. Some medical doctors use the regeneration technologies that low level light therapy (LLLT), now called photobiomodulation (PBM), but most do not.

The cause of this lack of utilization of technology is fairly common when a large, classical industry controls the flow of technology from the lab to the clinic.

The drug companies have had hundreds of failed drug trials but drugs for Alzheimer's, for the most part, work in mice, not people.

And the device makers are busy making and selling implantable devices, such as the Deep Brain Magnetic Stimulator (DBMS), which does amazing things for Parkinson's patients by eliminating their tremors.

Some studies have shown this technology can also help Alzheimer's patients, but it is not necessary to drill a hole in the skull and the brain to install a spark plug in the head, when shining a light on the cranium will do as well.

Unless your goal is revenue growth, where you are not measured on outcomes. Just sales, once FDA approved. Then the $100,000 device is much more valuable to promote than the less expensive photobiomodulation or low level light therapy.

It was on a trip to Vienna, Austria, three years ago, to meet medical device innovator Armin Bernhard, Ph.D., who, working with neurologist Elmar Weiler, Ph.D., had developed a therapy for reducing the discomfort of tinnitus (ringing in the ears).

The device was a foam pillow that you put your head in for twenty minutes, each day, and it helped you, without any drugs, drills, scalpels or implants. During their research they had also shown excellent results when used with a small number of patients with depression and dementia.

I could conceptualize how they might reduce a problem such as ringing in the ears. But Armin, with a Ph.D. in electrical engineering, had worked for Advanced Bionics, a company acquired by Boston Scientific for $750 million in 2005. He and

Elmar Weiler, Ph.D., a German neurologist, indicated the ability for cells that are dying to recover their health.

Their hypothesis was that the neurons need to sense a certain amount of electrical potential in their surrounding, or they die. As little as twenty minutes a day of the transcranial magnetic stimulation (TMS) would avoid the death of the neurons. And those on the borderline would recover! This I found startling. And exciting. As it turned out, there was evidence in the literature supporting this.

Transcranial Magnetic Stimulation (TMS) had been approved in the US for treating depression.

Armin referred to the need for electrical or magnetic energy in the brain as vitamins, indicating the brain needed a supplement to overcome an inadequacy of energy to sustain good health. When he used transcranial magnetic stimulation pulsed slowly (under 100 hertz), the cells stopped dying, and recovered!

"Do you mean that, when I see holes in the brain from the destruction of Alzheimer's, thought to be having to do with Amyloid plaque, that you can reverse the degeneration?"

"That is what it appears to us."

Vitamins. Like how vitamin C stops scurvy. Only, not in pill form. Directed energy, what DARPA had forecast in 1992 could be used in medicine.

A few months later I was fortunate to be introduced to Marvin Berman, Ph.D. a psychotherapist specializing in neurotherapy, also the president of the non-profit Quietmind Foundation in Philadelphia, PA.

Marvin had been doing studies with neurofeedback when he first learned of low level light therapy (LLLT) working on humans with Alzheimer's, from a physician in the United Kingdom who had been working with LLLT for years, and had developed several successful devices.

The first use by Dr. Dougal was to deter herpes 1 outbreaks on the lips, and the second to improve wrinkles in cosmetology, using near infrared light emitting diodes (LED's) in over the counter medical applications.

Dr. Dougal announced to the world that he had found a therapy, but did not yet have adequate studies published in refereed journals to justify the press releases that went around the world, in the minds of his peers.

Marvin Berman, a specialist in the use of neurofeedback, was involved in a trial trying it with Alzheimer's patients, when he learned of Dr. Dougal's work in the UK, and asked the spouse of one of his patients to consider it.

This was the original press release that caused awareness, and controversy. http://www.medgadget.com/2008/01/infrated_helment_to_stave_off_alzheimer-s.html

This led to the funding of the Quietmind Foundation's double blind, placebo controlled, study of Alzheimer's patients using Dr. Dougal's unique photobiomodulation device.

While expensive, and having a bit of a Rube Goldberg appearance, with some 1,000 LED's and 8 fans, it provided a powerful six minute therapy that had noticeable and measurable success in the treatment of Alzheimer's, over thirty days, and resulted in the double blind, placebo controlled study Dr. Berman presented at an Alzheimer's conference where he entertained inquiries from representatives of the National Institute of Health's Aging Division.

I tried on this helmet several times, and the results were astonishing on several levels. In 6 minutes of use (it times off after 6 minutes), I felt revitalized (as with taking caffeine, without the edge. As with most people who use it, I also experienced intensified visual recognition of colors and a surprising and never before 3D enhancement effect, when looking at plants in a garden. While other helmets help with dementia and Alzheimer's/TBI, none that I know of, or have ever used, have this effect. This helmet uses a frequency some 30 nanometers below 1100, whereas most others are at 660 and or 810 to 880.

Here are some of the results from the study presented: https://app.box.com/s/dr7366rvwejwt1jhcjv8ijxf45kjia7y by the Quietmind Foundation, using the Dougal helmet.

The Dougal helmet was also being used and tested in the UK, and in South Africa, and is still used and studied by Dr. Berman. All indications are it works, although there are less expensive devices that also work. Which works best has never been studied. That many appear to work with some success is recognized by the therapists using it and their patients, and the outcome of the double blind study, showing statistically significant results.

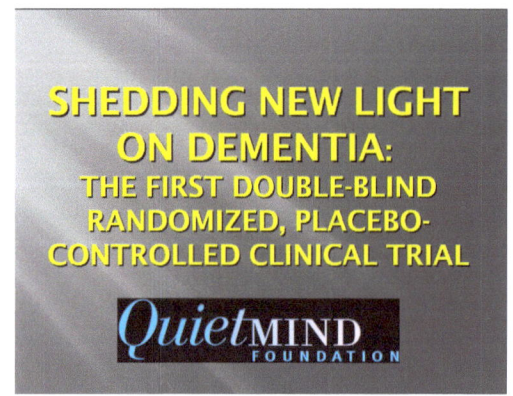

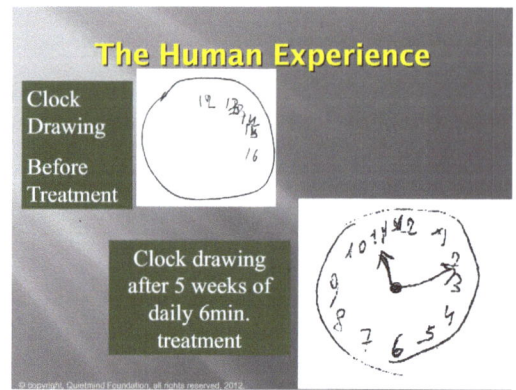

Dr. Berman and his medical colleagues on his Internal Review Board (IRB) then started experiments where the light therapy was combined with neurofeedback, specifically the type known as LORETA Z Score neurofeedback. It is considered a non-medical, brain training technology, but it does, in fact, have remarkable outcomes when used with Alzheimer's patients, TBI, ADHD, epilepsy, autism, and even Parkinson's. A review of the published literature will confirm this. I have provided many citations is the bibliography at the the end of this book.

LORETA Z SCORE NEUROFEEDBACK CAN DOUBLE COGNITIVE IMPROVEMENT

Dr. Berman found that, in the case of Alzheimer's patients, the combination of the two therapies resulted in each nearly doubling the effect of the other. Both were twice as good as either alone. However, the light therapy deterred the deadly tissue degeneration that erodes the brain and eventually can kill the patient. Without the low level light therapy (LLLT) the degeneration continues and destroys the brain cells. Even as the patient's memory recovers from neurofeedback tuning.

Whereas, the neurofeedback improves the brain wave output and can adjust the brainwave function so that those suffering from a degenerating brain can have their brainwaves adjusted back towards normal, improving both memory, personality and cognition. All measurably.

Both are essential. In sequence, light first, then neurofeedback. Every other day.

Dr. Berman and I spoke with Irving Rappaport, a well known patent attorney who at one time had served as the Chief Patent Counsel of Medtronic. And another time the Chief Patent Counsel at Apple, under Steve Jobs.

Irv thought the idea of patenting the combined therapy was very promising, and assisted us and a team of other patent attorneys on filing broad omnibus (able to generate many subsequent patents) filings that covered the many potential combination of neurologically beneficial light (or other energy, such as TUS, TMS, or PEMF), and other therapy with neurofeedback. I have provided some of the drawings so you can see how the tools to deliver the therapies to the clinic might work.

Stuart Hameroff, MD, an innovative anesthesiologist at the University of Arizona, also famous for his writings with Nobel laureate Roger Penrose, about the Science of Consciousness, had discovered as an outfall of his study of consciousness the astonishing result that ultrasound devices used to image the body, can have a therapeutic effect, if the imaging is done to the brain at the right frequency! Non-invasively.

This was the third energy source, first TMS, then PBM, and know transcranial ultrasound (TUS), that worked! We included these combinations in our patent filings, to enable the optimal combination therapy for each patient.

VIDEOS WORTH WATCHING

Many scientist trust their instincts when claiming this technology cannot possibly work. Evidence based medicine is inefficient when some evidence is dismissed, and not studied, and published.

[Photobiomodulation Lecture 2015 - Lew Lim, et al](#)
[Michael Hamblin, Ph.D. Harvard 1](#)
[Michael Weiner, the author of this book, October, 2015](#)
[ANIRBAN'S REMARKABLE DISCOVERY](#)

HOW DO WE KNOW THIS TECHNOLOGY WORKS?

The wars in Afghanistan and Iraq surprised Congress when thousands of soldiers came back suffering from Traumatic Brain Injury (TBI), and there was little understanding or therapy with which to treat it, PTSD, and other conditions.

Congress funded over $800 million in research at the Department of Defense (DOD and US Army) to solve the problem. They discovered the tremendous benefit that low level light therapy (LLLT), now also called photobiomodulation (PMB), has on improving the effects of Traumatic Brain Injury (TBI). I have provided links to both videos and scientific papers showing this.

Alzheimer's is very similar in how light therapy helps, but only one privately funded research institution in the US conducted research, and showed compelling evidence in 11 patients. This was presented in 2010 at an Alzheimer's conference attended by many leading scientists, including officials of the NIH. It was later presented to the Alzheimer's Association. For reasons not clear, the preference in both situations was to continue seeking pharmaceutical solutions, and ignore light therapy.

So the amount of scientific evidence is fairly limited, as far as double blind studies, which cost a great deal of money.

But the use of LLLT to treat many conditions is growing, and appears to work.

For over two years I have worked with the scientists and physicians who conducted the original study, and asked for additional studies to be funded. We asked the government agencies, we asked the Alzheimer's Association, and we asked industry, including most of the big device companies. No one to date has stepped up. Another Alzheimer's non-profit research organization has shown interest, and we are talking with them.

Other indications have also shown a correlation with several energy therapies and positive outcomes in Alzheimer's patients.

How astonishing, but consistent with the theory that the brain needs energy stimulation as much as it needs supplements to stay healthy. But medical science would have none of this without extensive evidence. This is the cause of many Catch 22's in medicine. You can't get the evidence if the folks in charge do not favor and fund the studies. So the evidence stacks up against you. And, you may be labeled a quack, and shunned by your peers.

Unless light therapy is tested for Alzheimer's, the public may get the $100,000 deep brain magnetic stimulators (DBMS) they do not need, ahead of the light therapy that they can afford. And LLLT would eliminate the hole drilled the skull, and brain, and the pacemaker like device in their chest.

TESTING THE HYPOTHESIS

I was on a conference call in early 2015 when I had trouble remembering how to do a conference call on my iPhone when also conferencing on my Panasonic home phone system. I wanted to go from the two people on the Panasonic, to the multiple people allowed on an iPhone conference.

I have used both for years, flawlessly, but I was stuck. I could not recall what to do. This happened several times, and then my memory recall of words, synonyms and names started to falter.

My business partner, Warren Woodford and I were co-authors of one of the best selling thesauruses on the market, the Word Finder thesaurus what was inside of WordStar, Microsoft Word, Claris and Symantec products in the 1980's (over 6 million copies sold or bundled). I could solve the Jumble puzzle most days in 1-2 minutes. When synonyms did not pop instantly out of my memory, and started to take 15-20 seconds, I knew something was wrong, and I knew what it likely was.

During my use of QEEG scans to understand what they did and how the neurofeedback technology adjust brainwaves non-invasively, while watching TV, it was discovered that I had had a Traumatic Brain Injury noticeable occluding my left

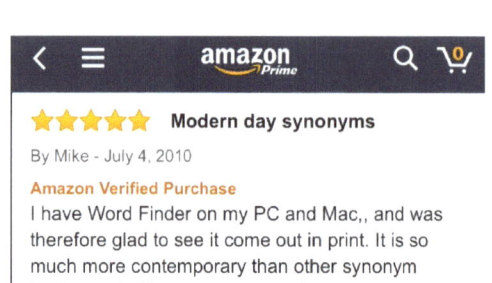

front temporal lobe. This was the result of my falling on the ice when I was fifteen, waking up in the hospital with a concussion. While I had hit the back of my head, on the right side, the injury wound up on the front, on the left, due to something they call coup contra coups, the bouncing of the brain upon impact.

I had learned that a person with TBI is <u>4-8 times more likely</u> to suffer early stage dementia…

And I had it!

I decided to take matters into my own hands.

I first had Dr. Berman refer me to a local neurotherapist expert in neurofeedback. To determine which parts of my brain most needed tuning, I had a quantitative electroencephalogram (QEEG), which enabled LORETA Z score biofeedback. I had this therapy twice a week. It used a shower cap like device with 19 electrodes recording, and a clip on your ear.

Warren recommended a supplier of a handheld, inexpensive, infrared light with 120 LED's at one of the effective frequencies, available on the Internet (from theledman.com).

I purchased it, and commenced shining it on my head every morning for ten minutes two minutes over the injury, two minutes over each temple, two minutes on the crown of my head, and two minutes in the back of the head there the skull meets the neck. I used it every day, although some makers of infrared suggest every other day. As it turns out, we now believe that using it just in advance of the neurofeedback is optimal, for several reasons. My therapy closely approximated this.

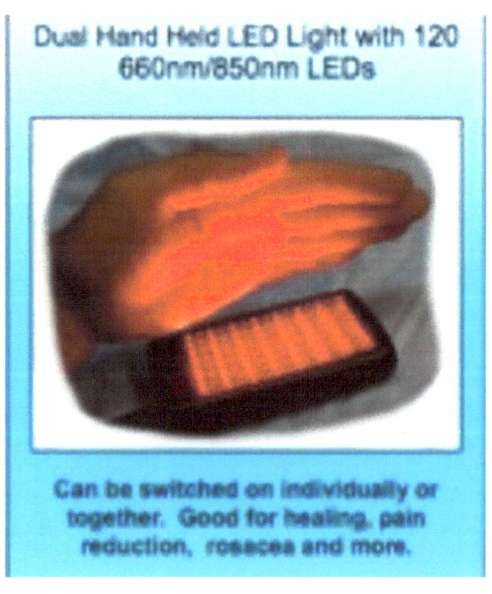

Within six weeks my memory was fully restored! No more lapses or confusion. My brain scans fully supported my feeling of recovery. And they appeared to my therapist and her colleagues remarkably fast in changing. I attribute this to the use of light therapy.

I can provide a link to the full study over six weeks, and I now have it showing over a year, with continual improvement of other areas of the brain. A chart of the six weeks of scans will be shown in just a few pages.

You would need to understand how the scans are plotted, but effectively, the closer the center line, the better, as it represents the norm of people with normal brain patterns.

The further away, the less optimized are the brainwaves.

I used two devices during my first year of therapy. First a 120 LED unit at 660, and when I lost it on a trip, I then purchased two dual frequency unit, as the 880 nanometer was helping a friend who had suffered from debilitating back pain from a fractured disk, and the light (at 880) made a life-changing improvement.

My technical experts believe that light in the 800 to 830 nanometer near-infrared (NIR) range, is best for Alzheimer's. TheLEDman.com will special order an 830 nanometer device for just a few dollars extra. It is not sold for any specific medical purpose. It is a hobbyist device. But it works. I will be buying the much more powerful Brain Buffer device, for shorter light therapy sessions, as soon as it is available, later this year (see the addendum in the back of this book).

How light therapy actuates cellular healing is indicated in this slide from Michael Hamblin, Ph.D.s work on light therapy:

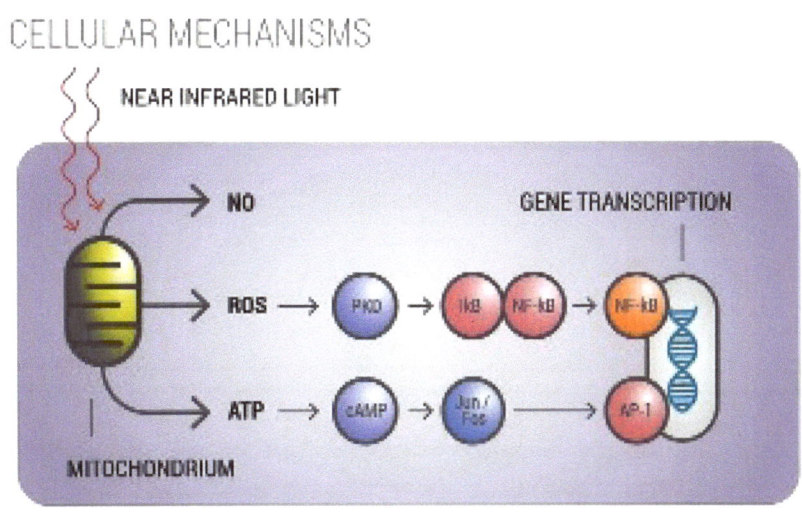

Reference: "Basic Photomedicine", Ying-Ying Huang, Pawel Mroz. and Michael R. Hamblin, Harvard Medical School.

Much information on the mechanism of action of light can be found on the web and some key links can be viewed at http://lumineu.com/science.

My memory and QEEG scores have been stable for over a year, but the results of the neurofeedback is now that the lines of the right side have compressed again, closer to the bottom, which is the desired outcome. The sessions are also a great deal of fun, and quite fascinating.

The system compares your brainwaves in multiple areas of the brain to the normative database, which is divided into age groups, gender, and right or left handedness. You are compared to your peer group and the system detects where your brainwaves need adjustment. Software from Applied Neuroscience then is used to develop the brain tuning goals for the neurofeedback sessions.

This is my brain scan after only 6 weeks of twice weekly neurofeedback training, accompanied by the use of the red LED light held next to my scalp, ten minutes each day. Ideally before the neurofeedback, and before evening not to keep me up.

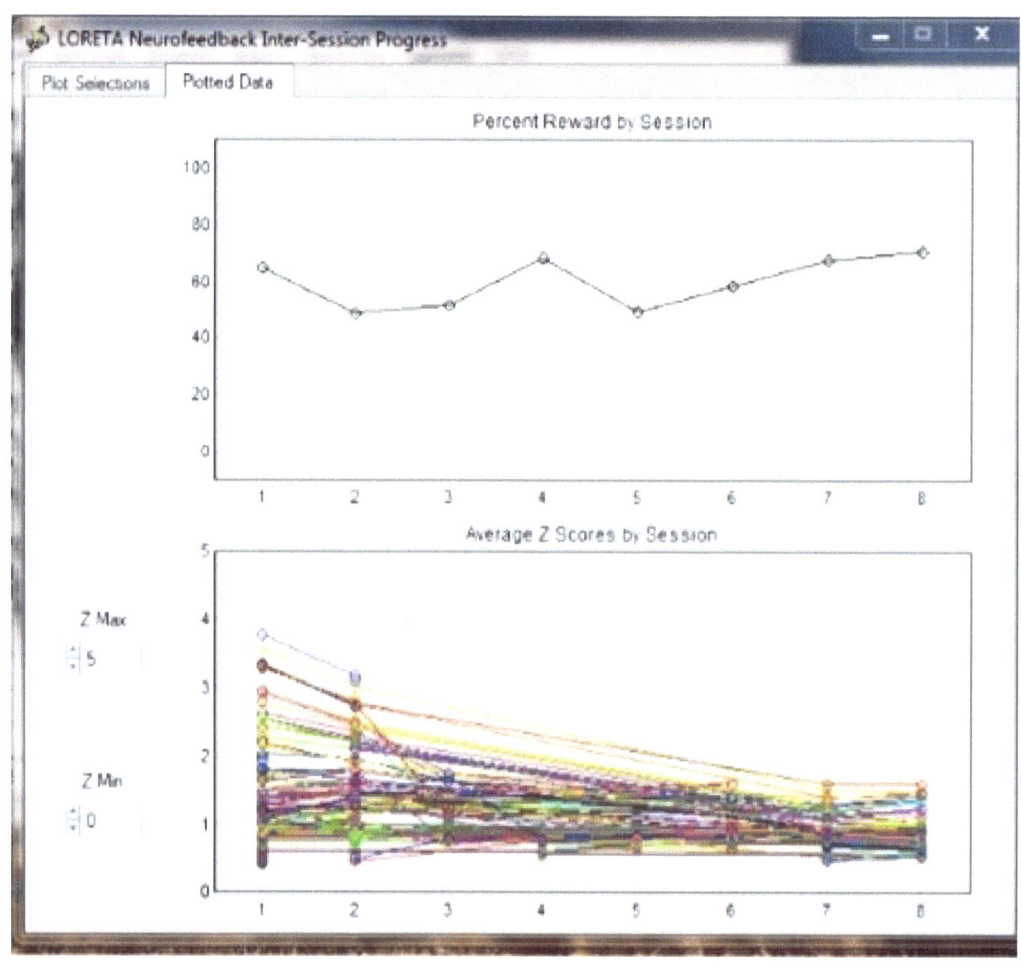

I watch television while electrodes on my head, are listening to your brainwaves in real time. And the system gives you feedback which your brain processes without your having to do anything but watch tv.

As any of the brainwaves veer away from the norm for that area, the system changes the color saturation and audio of the television, so it goes from color to black and white, and the audio goes off.

The brain attempts to find a way to fix this, before you know what to think or do, and the video and audio return to normal when this happens, in a second or two. Over the course of a twenty minute session over 300 instances of this training occur (appliedneuroscience.com).

Which does remarkable things to the brain and memory, and can work with anyone, even an Alzheimer's patient.

In my case, I watched Seinfeld, catching up on episodes that I missed, and enjoying those I had not seen for years. It is a pleasant experience and works remarkably well.

The feeling of your brain slowing down in real time and not retrieving what you need is a very bothersome affair. It scared me. The fact that this therapy and a referral to a competent therapist turned it around, that quickly, and easily, has spurred me on that much more assertively to get industry to adopt this miraculous technology. And to add light therapy with it.

Even though the amount of money that can be made solving Alzheimer's is enormous, folks in industry understand and obey the unwritten rules of business.

Taking a risk on an innovation that sounds different than the norm, and might make less explosive jumps in revenue perceived per procedure, and profits, than what they are used to, today, is a powerful sedative to innovation in the big companies.

So powerful that I decided to write this book, and provide you with the evidence of the success, first at the level needed by a person with a loved one with the problem, or having memory problems themselves.

To the industry executives who are complacent and slow moving, I offer this bit of data.

1 million pacemakers are implanted annually, and this generates north of $10 billion annually in highly profitable dollars, and generates a market cap of over $100 billion, amongst just the three companies that dominate that industry.

40 million people have Alzheimer's.

PBM IS NOT THE ONLY THERAPY - IT MAY BE THE BEST.

Photobiomodulation is the most studied and reported on that I am familiar with, in stopping and deterring Alzheimer's. But there are other potentials, both non-invasive and invasive.

It appears to be the most studies and the most effective, but anyone interested in how to get energy into an energy starved brain should also investigate transcranial ultrasound (TUS), transcranial magnetic stimulation (TMS), transcranial pulsed electromagnetic fields (PEMF), and other potential energy and delivery methods.

What is unique is that something on the market and safe, infrared light, works, safely and effectively. It is not a drug with unknown dangers. The NIH should step up to the plate, and fund studies. They are a very large organization with their own protocols and procedures. I am working with them to explore this opportunity. Same with the many foundations involved with Alzheimer's research funding. Many are stuck in non-innovative methods of looking at new innovation.

It is bothersome that something with this much promise is not being more urgently explored and pursued, as if time were not of the essence. That is the purpose of my writing this little book. Illumination may help.

EVIDENCE THAT LIGHT THERAPY HELPS PEOPLE WITH TBI

Improved Cognitive Function After Transcranial, Light-Emitting Diode ...
www.ncbi.nlm.nih.gov/.../PMC31042...
National Center for Biotechnology Information
by MA Naeser - 2011 - Cited by 95 - Related articles
Objective: Two chronic, traumatic brain injury (TBI) cases, where cognition improved following treatment with red and near-infrared light-emitting diodes (LEDs), ...
Can light therapy help the brain? >VA study with 160 Gulf War ...
www.research.va.gov/.../sprin...
Veterans Health Administration Office of Research an...
Mar 31, 2015 - Following up on promising results from pilot work, researchers at the VA Boston Healthcare System are testing the effects of light therapy on brain function in Veterans with Gulf War Illness. Veterans in the study wear a helmet lined with light-emitting diodes that apply red and ...
TBI: Mild Traumatic Brain Injury Symptoms | Concussions | Mild Head ...
www.traumaticbraininjury.com/symptoms-of-tbi/mild-tbi-symptoms/
Other Symptoms Associated with Mild TBI. Nausea; Loss of smell; Sensitivity to light and sounds; Mood changes; Getting lost or confused; Slowness in thinking.
New Study Discovers Near-Infrared Light Therapy ... - PR Newswire
www.prnewswire.com/.../new-study-discovers-near-infrared-light-therapy-nilt-effecti...
Aug 21, 2015 - 21, 2015 /PRNewswire/ -- New Study Discovers Near-Infrared Light Therapy (NILT) Effectively Treats Traumatic Brain Injury (TBI)...
Traumatic Brain Injury & Light Therapy - YouTube

Video for tbi and light▶ 5:21
https://www.youtube.com/watch?v=15lRFTqkYCg
Mar 4, 2014 - Uploaded by In Light Hyperbarics
Traumatic Brain Injury & Light Therapy. In Light Hyperbarics ... Can near-infrared energy reach the brain ...

Low-level light therapy for traumatic brain injury
www2.massgeneral.org/.../faculty-hamblin-research-lo...
Massachusetts General Hospital
There are no approved therapies for traumatic brain injury (TBI) despite an ... Transcranial application of near-infrared laser or LED light is non-invasive, ...
Recovering from Mild Traumatic Brain Injury | BrainLine Military
www.brainlinemilitary.org › Military TBI Topics › Brain Injury Symptoms
Recovering from Mild Traumatic Brain Injury (MTBI)): A Handbook of Hope for ... You may feel a heightened sensitivity to light and may even need to wear your ...
Treatment of Post-TBI Fatigue with Light Therapy - Icahn School of ...
icahn.mssm.edu/...traumatic-brain-injury.../treatment-of-post-tbi-fatigue-with-light-th...
Treatment of Post-TBI Fatigue with Light Therapy. Fatigue is a common problem after TBI that affects up to 80% of individuals with TBI (far more than the general ...
Bright Light Therapy Improves Sleep, Cognition in Mild TBI - Medscape
www.medscape.com/viewarticle/805547
Medscape
Jun 10, 2013 - BALTIMORE, Maryland — Bright light therapy may improve sleep and aid recovery after mild traumatic brain injury (TBI), new research hints.
New Study Discovers Near-Infrared Light Therapy (NILT) Effectively ...
www.tbi.care/.../new-study-discovers-near-infrared-light-therapy-nilt-effectively-treat...
Aug 21, 2015 - The exciting news is that NIR light, in the 10-15W range at 810 nm and 980 nm, can safely and effectively treat chronic symptoms of TBI.

HOW AND WHERE TO GET THE THERAPY

Neurofeedback is available in almost every city. I suggest visiting the web site of the non-profit biofeedback certification association, BCIA,org, and looking for a therapist near you. Call them up and find out if they provide LORETA Z score neurofeedback. Find out their cost and decide which therapist to see. The therapist will perform a QEEG scan and advise you of the neurofeedback sessions, which if you can afford them, will cost. Go twice weekly.

Then you need to find a near infrared light source. Here there are many on the market, from as little as $200 to as much as $10,000 or more.

None will be sold as for use with Alzheimer's, until such time as a manufacturer goes through the process of FDA approval. So you need to power and frequency requirements.

You have to determine if you believe this story, because you can only buy these lights for innocuous purposes, relief of muscle pain, relaxation, etc.

Actually, the scientific literature is filled with information on the way that infrared light improves the output of ATP, the fuel of the cell, in the mitochondria in each of your cells. And it up regulates other factors, nitric oxide (NO), vascular endothelial growth factors (VEGF), and much more.

Studies show that the best frequencies are in the 800 to 830 nanometer range.

However, Dr. Berman's study was with the Dougal helmet, in the 1070 nanometer range. That device put out a lot of energy, all over the head and over the eyes, and only needed a 6 minute session. But that device costs around $8,000 and is not available for sale in the US, although it can be obtained through an IRB study through the Quietmind Foundation.

I have listed in an addendum several that range from several hundred dollars up to $3,000, and their parameters. They all should be helpful. Which is better, and what the price to value ratios are, I do not know.

There are also clinicians who may have infrared devices they can treat you with on a per visit basis. This may be helpful if you wish to try these technologies before you commit. Not all infrared lights are the same frequency. I have had success using 660 nanometer, in the visible red light range. Above 780 is near infrared, and you cannot see the light. 810-830 appear the most tested and successful frequencies, but 1072, the Dougal frequency, should not be excluded.

Heating is not what you are looking for, in fact, you want to avoid lamps that get very warm to hot. The effect is not thermal. It is photonic. So I suggest using one of the devices shown, which fall into the operational range. It is my estimation that pulsing is not essential, although some vendors consider pulsing really important.

One of the leading scientists in photobiomodulation, who has done much of the research on traumatic brain injury (TBI), is Michael Hamblin, Ph.D. at the Wellman Institute at Harvard.

I found a video interview with him on the Internet which is extremely informative and answers many questions. I strongly recommend that you watch it, as it will answer many questions for everyone from lay persons to knowledgeable scientists and physicians.

Michael Hambrich, Ph.D. at Harvard and Mass General Video on LLLT

https://www.youtube.com/watch?v=wAW8Fvg-TJQ

He also has a paper we recommend: Role of Low-Level Laser Therapy in Neurorehabilitation

http://www.ncbi.nlm.nih.gov/pmc/articles/PMC3065857/

Hamblin speaks here to TBI, but the technology is essentially the same as we are using for Alzheimer's, with the exception that we find that combining neurofeedback with light therapy measurably increases cognitive results, enough to startle many family members when a loved one is treated with both. For both Alzheimer's, TBI, and, even Parkinson's!

ONE OF HAMBLIN'S PAPERS

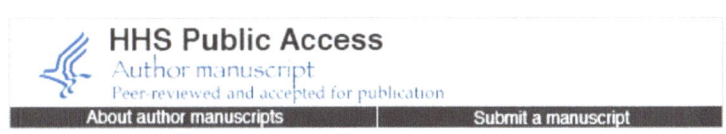

PM R. Author manuscript; available in PMC 2011 Dec 1.
Published in final edited form as:
PM R. 2010 Dec; 2(12 Suppl 2): S292–S305.
doi: 10.1016/j.pmrj.2010.10.013

PMCID: PMC3065857
NIHMSID: NIHMS281845

Role of Low-Level Laser Therapy in Neurorehabilitation

Javad T. Hashmi, MD, Ying-Ying Huang, MD, Bushra Z. Osmani, MD, Sulbha K. Sharma, PhD, Margaret A. Naeser, PhD, LAc, and Michael R. Hamblin, PhD

Author information ▶ Copyright and License information ▶

Abstract

Go to: ☑

This year marks the 50th anniversary of the discovery of the laser. The development of lasers for medical use, which became known as low-level laser therapy (LLLT) or photobiomodulation, followed in 1967. In recent years, LLLT has become an increasingly mainstream modality, especially in the areas of physical medicine and rehabilitation. At first used mainly for wound healing and pain relief, the medical applications of LLLT have broadened to include diseases such as stroke, myocardial infarction, and degenerative or traumatic brain disorders. This review will cover the mechanisms of LLLT that operate both on a cellular and a tissue level. Mitochondria are thought to be the principal photoreceptors, and increased adenosine triphosphate, reactive oxygen species, intracellular calcium, and release of nitric oxide are the initial events. Activation of transcription factors then leads to expression of many protective, anti-apoptotic, anti-oxidant, and pro-proliferation gene products. Animal studies and human clinical trials of LLLT for indications with relevance to neurology, such as stroke, traumatic brain injury, degenerative brain disease, spinal cord injury, and peripheral nerve regeneration, will be covered.

Information on neurofeedback can be found at www.appliedneuroscience.com. However, we suspect this may also play a role.
http://www.sciencedaily.com/releases/2011/08/110811083820.htm

Additional background can be found at the www.quietmindfdn.org.

Results of their double blind, placebo controlled study can be found here:

https://app.box.com/s/dr7366rvwejwt1jhcjv8ijxf45kjia7y

Other publications on the effects of light therapy and neurofeedback can be found at these links:

https://app.box.com/files/0/f/5342905953/Clinical_Data

Presentations by the Quietmind Foundation to the NIH and to the Alzheimer's Association, and other evidence can be found at this link:

https://app.box.com/s/eckoa4ot946itugwjc6r61n1x9mvlnz0

Lumineu, Inc. has a web site with a great deal of useful information (lumineu.-com). Additional data can be viewed at https://app.box.com/s/77b-szm2x57zm1ukwsdjitygcqnxxuti5, and noothera.com.

Lumineu acquired the patents of NooThera, AND is planning clinical trials for an automated therapy device that provides both light therapy and neurofeedback. It can be used daily in the clinic or at home, quite affordably, seeing the therapist and neurologist perhaps quarterly instead of several times per week. If you are interested in having someone participated in the clinical trials, please write to me at phasemike@gmail.com, and I will let you know if there are trials being planned near you (there are both patient sponsored trials and foundation sponsored, that is, paid).

This technology has the potential to reduce the cost of therapy for each one million people from $50 billion per year down to $10 billion, and eliminating the need to transport patients to the clinic several times per week: https://app.box.-com/s/77bszm2x57zm1ukwsdjitygcqnxxuti5. Investors may wish to contact the company if they wish to invest. (I am an investor in this company.)

Those wishing to make tax deductible contributions can contact the Quietmind Foundation (www.quietmindfdn.org).

Those wishing to support my efforts to get the word out and change the industry can buy the book, or refer it to friends. Or visit https://www.gofundme.com/stop-Alzheimer-s.

Useful links on photobiomodulation and neurofeedback can be found in the addendum.

HOW TO TREAT ALZHEIMER'S AND TRAUMATIC BRAIN INJURY (TBI)

I am not offering medical advice. You should turn to your physician for that, when treating any cognitive disorder or degenerating disease.

However, this book, by relating my personal experience and much published research, may arm you with what is needed to help your physician overcome the lack of funding for innovative alternatives, and the industry complacency. This is what is needed to stop the tragic pandemic. A sense of urgency, and interest in new solutions that work, versus old ones, that have not.

I have been working on the business plan and patents to get this vital technology onto the market so lives and families can be saved. Having worked for several years, at great personal cost and effort, by myself and a dozen colleagues.

It appears that, while this technology can get into the clinic in less than two years, with full FDA approval and astonishing affordability, it may not. Because the industry is not competitive in the way it could, or should be.

With the issue that 30,000 patients per year die in the US alone, and they are replaced by the newly diagnosed take their place at the beginning of a five to twenty year decline into hell itself. Those are the statistics that occur in the US with the population of 5 million Alzheimer's patients, and another several million with other forms of dementia.

WHY THIS BOOK?

I decided to write this book with three specific goals:

1) to educate the public that there is a solution, how I obtained the therapy, and how it worked for me, and others. And to point to the preponderance of evidence that is in the published literature, and not in the clinic, other than in limited clinical trials.

2) To illustrate the inefficiency of industry, government and foundations that can turn a blind eye to this potential, and not fund clinical trials while pharmaceutical alternatives are funded, and for the most part, have not worked.

3) As an industry innovator and networker, I believe one of the device companies can make a good return on investment by pursuing this technology, and the broad patents that have been filed. So can accredited investors and family offices. I hope to meet you if this is of interest. Or call me at (239) 603-6446.

WHERE TO GET THE TECHNOLOGY AND HOW TO USE IT

The Quietmind Foundation is the only organization I am aware of conducting clinical trials on the combination of low level light therapy and neurofeedback.

There are dozens of products already on the market, deemed safe by FDA as Class II medical devices, that are sold for purposes from pain relief to muscle relaxation. Those in the frequency bands that work for treating Alzheimer's are available, but cannot be sold for that purpose, because the industry has not decided to invest the money for FDA approval. It could take a study of perhaps 100 people in a trial that might be as short as 90 days.

Studies, including those included in the addendum and links in this book, indicate that infrared devices in the range of 800 to 830 nanometers, near infrared, beyond the red light range to where the lights do not emit visible light, are most effective at stimulating the brain to revitalize neurons, increasing the nerve pads, dendrites and synapses in the brain at rapid rates after a short exposure to the light at those frequencies. However, 1072 has also had significant success. The public health crisis cannot take the time to determine which is best, when both work. We need to get the therapy into the clinics in the same way that using Vitamin C stopped scurvy, and washing hands reduced infectious disease. People are dying while healthcare leaders dither.

Watch out for heating. Some systems do not put forth much heat, and others put forth a great deal. Most used to treat the skin surface do not. If the lamp makes your scalp warm, or uncomfortable, discontinue use.

I will show you where you can get a dozen for prices between under $200 and up to several thousand dollars, at one of the frequency bands that has shown to work, and have been evaluated for power, frequency and heat output, as safe for use by humans.

Red light, in the 660 to 670 nanometer range, also seems to work fairly well. That is what I used to overcome my memory loss from TBI, before I learned about the higher frequencies.

Marvin Berman, Ph.D., and president of the Quietmind Foundation, has uses a 1072 device, made in the UK, which has a very powerful output and a short dosing time (6 minutes), which has a more powerful and noticeable effect (you see enhanced colors and 3D after usage, and feel quite stimulated). However that device is available, only through the Foundation as part of their IRB approved clinical trials. Other devices are available, but are not sold for use for treating Alzheimer's. Studies are needed. A list of devices on the market that offer the same features as those that have worked in clinical trials is available at the end of this book.

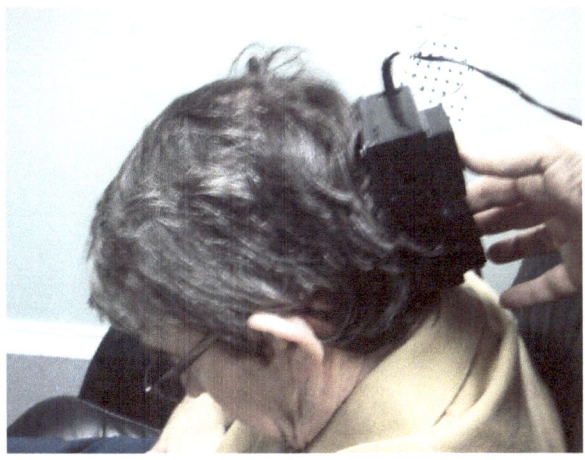

A Parkinson's patient with an unsuccessful DBMS implant being given light therapy in the base of the skull with a custom built 1072 device.
above: patient getting treatment for Parkinson's. The patient and therapist reported reduction in tremors. See the quietmindfdn.org web site.

These devices were the ones studied in the double blind, placebo controlled study done by the QMF Foundation, under IRB approved studies, in 2010, and reported to the NIH (2009)and the Alzheimer's Association (in 2015), who they hope will fund additional studies. Funders continue to hope for a drug solution, versus non-invasive therapies. This is the fundamental drawback.

A popular and relatively affordable device is the Neuro from Vielight, a company in Canada who makes a helmet with four laser diode modules that fit over key areas of the brain where neuronal switching takes place, and much early stage Alzheimer's seems to occur. The Neuro sells for $1,500, although some

When combined with neurofeedback, which is highly recommended, it is best to use the light shortly before the neurofeedback session. It is also advisable to eat before the neurofeedback session. It is not yet known if the light helps Alzheimer's degeneration or just enhances neurofeedback, but the therapy has merit. A more powerful light for Alzheimer's therapy should also be considered.

At this time the optimal neurofeedback, known as LORETA Z Score neurofeedback, is available only through neurotherapists. They are trained in how to read a special brain scan called a QEEG (quantitative electroencephalogram), a map of your brainwaves, and compare it to a normative database collected over many years, and organized by gender, age, and left of right handedness.

They use sophisticated software, such as Neuroguide from Applied Neuroscience, Inc., or BrainMaster, which provides feedback to the patient that retunes their brainwaves.

Lumineu, Inc. has filed patents on an automated device that combines both laser light, and automated neurotherapy, that can be monitored and changed remotely. This can reduce the cost of twice weekly out patient therapy.

This therapy has been shown in many studies to help many indications, but is not considered medicine. This is lucky for the consumer, as many trained practitioners provide the service, which is considered training, versus medicine. However, if anyone sold this as a therapy for Alzheimer's, depression, ADHD, Parkinson's, etc., they risk violating the law for offering a medical device or therapy. So Catch 22 stands in the way of both therapies.

Even though both work without contraindication or any known negatives.

It just can't be offered to the public until some company is willing to spend the money to comply with the FDA rules and regs. Which so far no company has been willing to do.

You will have to check with your insurance company about whether or not they will pay for neurofeedback. The sessions needed perhaps twice a week tend to range in the $100 to $150 each range. And the Alzheimer's patient has to be transported to and from the therapist's office. I have heard that ADHD, which neurofeedback can resolve, instead of drug dependency, is covered by some insurance plans, in at least some states. Check with a therapist.

What should a family member due when such a technology appears to work, is not offered or being investigated by industry, and patients risk loss of memory and eventual death from a deadly disease?

What I did, and cannot recommend that you do, unless you have consulted with your physician, was to pick a light source, purchase it (some can be bought with a 30 day money back guarantee if not satisfied), and start using it twice daily, for 10 to 20 minutes. Holding it against the location of injury, or if not known, at the recommended top, temples, back of the neck, and frontal lobes.

For Alzheimer's I suggest several minutes over each temple, then on the top of the head, the back of the skull where it meets the neck, and each of the two frontal lobes, left and right. For about 2-4 minutes at each location, depending on the device. Most require about 20 minutes per session, but some of them require less time, such as the Brain Buffer and the Dougal helmet (6 minutes each), neither of which are on the market in the US, but may be through trials such as undertaken by the Quietmind Foundation. The Brain Buffer will be available for brain stimulation, as a non-medical device. It has the desired power and frequency. Clinical trials using more powerful and industrial strength devices (also more expensive), are being proposed, and need to be funded.

Neurofeedback sessions are optimally done shortly after the light therapy, or the next day, as this helps prepare the brain for the plasticity that neurofeedback induces, through watching videos on an LCD screen connected to the computer.

Both the light therapy and neurofeedback will usually show progress in the patient within several sessions. However, while neurofeedback and light therapy each almost double the output of the other, when combined, neurofeedback appears to retune the brain and generate improved cognition. Light therapy appears to increase the growth and health of the neurons, resulting in growth of nerve pads, dendrites and synapses. And stop the deadly degeneration.

Light therapy also appears to stop or deter the neurodegeneration and stabilize the destruction. So if you can only afford or obtain one, it is light therapy that will sustain life and reduce damage. The optimal solution are the two, combined. But if you can only use one, get the light first and use it regularly.

For optimal results, use both. The same appears true for TBI, where a great many more studies exist, funded mostly by the Department of Defense. No vendor we are aware of has stepped up to funding an FDA clinical trial to prove safety and efficacy, and then sell a device.

For other issues, such as **ADHD**, neurofeedback can resolve issues, including the need for drugs such as Ritalin, even in your children. Consult a local neurotherapist. You can find one at bcia.org, the non-profit accreditation organization.

There are also neurotherapists member another organization called ISNR (isnr.org)

A call to Applied Neuroscience (appliedneuroscienc.com) or Brainmasters, can provide referrals to practitioners near you.

At this moment I am not aware of organizations, other than the Quietmind Foundation, who provide the combined therapy.

So I recommend acquiring a near infrared light, self-administering it, and arranging for a visit to a neurotherapist for a QEEG scan.

There are some companies who may offer combined devices for general brain health, and not for Alzheimer's therapy, which will have to be provided by an MD after FDA approval. But if a device is on the market with both LLLT and neurofeedback, it may be very useful to examine if you have someone in need of treatment for Alzheimer's or TBI.

Studies have shown that there are several effective frequencies that work to slow and deter degeneration of Alzheimer's and TBI, but which is best is not clear.

Some have had success with read light at 660 nanometers, and there some at higher and lower frequencies (630 and 670), there is a consensus held by many that 810 is very effective, and 830 is not far from it. And then Dr. Dougal in the UK and Dr. Berman in Philadelphia have worked with success at the frequencies near 1070.

Powers vary, depth of penetration varies, and recommend time of therapy varies. Prices also vary quite a bit.

Some devices are built for clinical use, to a higher durability and industrial standard, and carry a commensurately higher price. If you are getting this for a single or family at home use, you may do well with any of the models.

Frequency, power, heating, and size are all factors you may wish to consider.

The best information is to list devices which either have been tested with Alzheimer's and / or TBI patients, or devices that have the same frequency and power ratings, and allow you to determine which you feel will meet your needs.

These devices are not on the market, at least as yet, for the treatment of Alzheimer's. They meet some other need, perhaps pain reduction, muscle relaxation, skin therapy, hair therapy, et al. And they are sold only for that purpose. So, if you decide to acquire a device and try it, you will need to do so at your own risk. If the device is already considered safe for human use, on or near the skin, shining it on your head is quite likely safe. But any one selling it for use as a therapy Alzheimer's is violating the law, unless it has FDA approval for that purpose.

Most units are offered for sale for a stated use, and some may note that these devices have been used experientially for one malady or another, and worked, to some extent.

Those who suffer from Parkinson's may also find these technologies helpful. However, if you have a Deep Brain Magnetic Stimulator (DBMS), do not use any light on the top of the head, as there have been reports of severe nightmares occurring. Best to place the light at the base of the skull where it meets the neck, if you have a DBMS device, particularly if you are one of the 20% of recipients who are not fortunate to experience the full control of tremors that a successful DBMS provides.

Is it fair that we are so close in the laboratory, with this technology, used in human clinical trial since before 2009, and that it is still not on the market? The studies showed statistically significant effectiveness, with no contraindications.

30,000 people a month die from Alzheimer's after many year of suffering, in the United States, alone.

This is main reason I am writing this book. To get the facts out.

NORM DOIDGE'S AMAZING BOOKS ON LIGHT THERAPY

Here is an excerpt from Norm Doidge, MD's excellent book, the Brain that Changes Itself. It is a great story of the advances of light therapy, ignored by most of the medical community for the traditional therapies. Here is a short sample: https://app.box.com/files/0/f/6356910553/1/f_51747972581

A later book, the Brain's Way of Healing, has updated information and light therapy doing amazing things for patients that traditional medicine fears.
https://read.amazon.com/kp/embed?
asin=B000QCTNIW&asin=B000QCTNIW&preview=newtab&linkCode=kpe&ref_=cm_sw_r_kb_dp_tGpMxbHVNNG0S

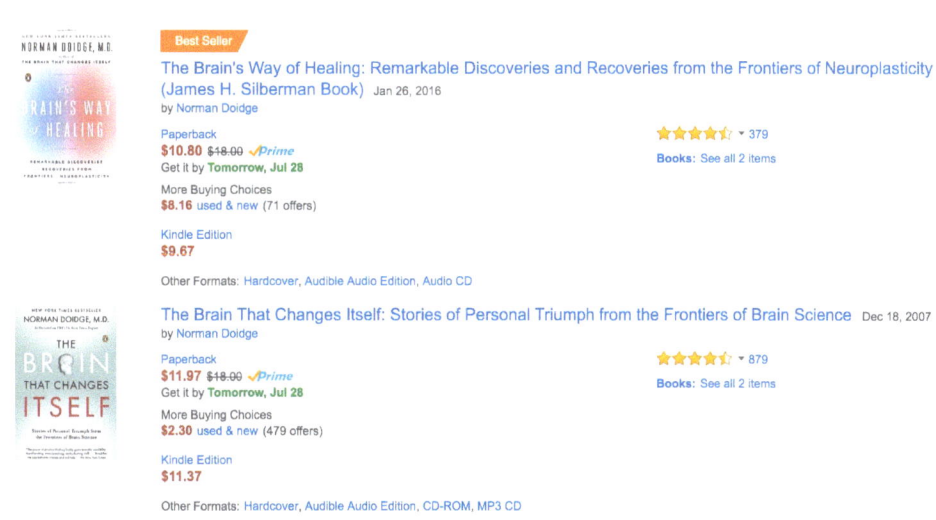

LUMINEU, INC.

Lumineu, a company commercializing the combined therapy, currently designing a home therapy device and planning clinical trials and FDA studies, has patents that teach a method for automated daily therapy of both light and neurofeedback, based on the input of the neurotherapist after they examine a QEEG scan.

The Lumineu device then uses the program that is selected for several weeks or months, by the neurologist and neurotherapist, until the patient revisits the therapies, and the daily sessions can be changed to work on other areas of the brain and brainwaves. The device also provides the low level light therapy (LLLT), or photobiomodulation (PBM) as it is now called.

First US patients treated with noninvasive focused ultrasound for Parkinson's disease

September 2, 2015

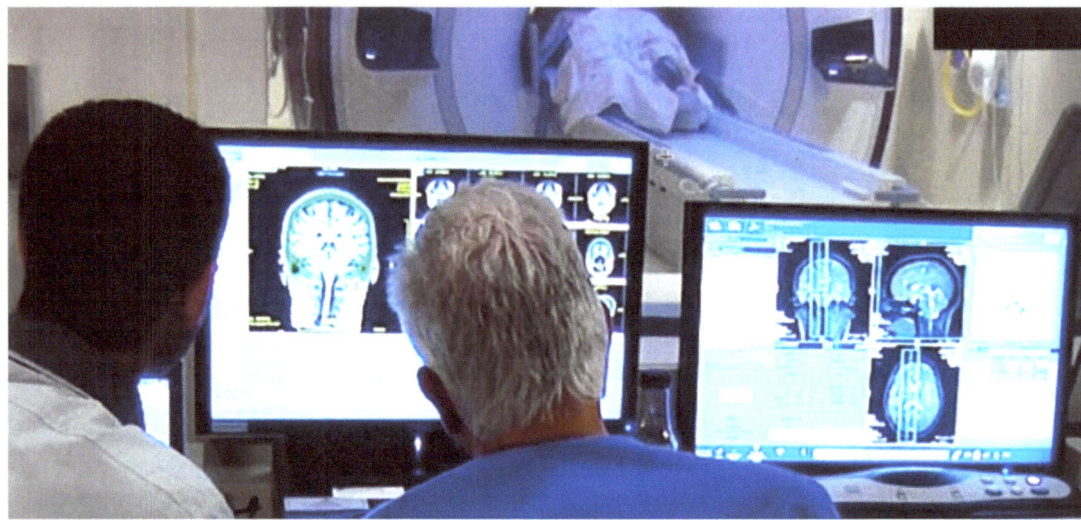

University of Maryland medical doctors monitor focused ultrasound treatment for essential tremor, guided by magnetic resonance imaging (MRI) (credit: University of Maryland School of Medicine)

Researchers at the University of Maryland have performed the first focused ultrasound treatments on a deep structure within the brain related to Parkinson's disease* called the globus pallidus.

These treatments are part of international pilot studies of 40 patients assessing the feasibility, safety, and preliminary efficacy of focused ultrasound treatments for Parkinson's disease, guided by magnetic resonance imaging (MRI).

The researchers are using MRI to help them guide ultrasound waves through the intact skin and skull to reach the globus pallidus part of the brain. If successful, focused ultrasound could offer an alternative approach for certain patients with Parkinson's disease who have failed medical therapy or become disabled from medication-induced dyskinesia (tremor). To date, seven patients in Korea and one patient in Canada have been treated in studies.

The new Parkinson's procedure

LIGHT THERAPY (LLLT OR PBM) AND PARKINSON'S

https://www.google.com/search?q=LIGHT+THERAPY+AND+PARKINSON%27S&oq=LIGHT+THERAPY+AND+PARKINSON%27S&aqs=chrome..69i57j0l2j69i61l3.4012j0j4&sourceid=chrome&ie=UTF-8

ULTRASOUND AND PARKINSON'S

http://www.kurzweilai.net/first-us-patients-treated-with-noninvasive-focused-ultrasound-for-parkinsons-disease

How astonishing, but consistent with the theory that the brain needs energy stimulation as much as it needs supplements to stay healthy.

WHY ARE THESE TECHNOLOGIES NOT ON THE MARKET FROM MAJOR COMPANIES?

This certainly is a logical question. To understand the limitation in the medical device industry and why it has not yet acted. you have to understand how very large, profitable companies process information.

Big companies plan their product lines years in advance, and are regulated by how much risk there is for an insider on staff to pitch a new technology. The pioneering company then needs to commit or raise the needed capital to do the studies, get the FDA approval, get insurance payer approval, and generate the working capital to visit clinicians and persuade them to try the technology.

The same is true of most venture capitalists. The main market for a company with a bold new innovation is acquisition by one of the giants. If a technology such asa non-invasive photobiomodulation device is not sought by the big companies, for whatever reason, the likelihood of VC investment is greatly diminished.

Then there are the perceived borders. Drug companies are expert on pharmaceuticals, and don't usually dabble in devices.. And vice versa. There are crossover products, such as drug coated stents, and implantable insulin pumps. And Abbott has venture more and more into the device space, particularly with the recent acquisition of St. Jude Medical (not the hospital, the device maker) for $30 billion. GSK has a venture fund to pursue electroceuticals.

The bigger drawback is, who is going to take the risk to go from the dozens of experiments and anecdotes, and spend the required $10 to $20 million on the double blind, placebo controlled clinical trial study needed to convince physicians, scientists and insurance payers that this technology works in rigorous studies? More is then needed for FDA trials of the actual device proposed for sale.

It is a Catch 22 scenario.

Hence, this book is to get the word out, and a crowd funding site in development for this pioneering company, Lumineu, that I helped several scientists, physicians and psychotherapists start.

Two years ago we designed pioneering patents for a revolution in medicine, including automating the home therapy, so millions of Alzheimer's do not have to be transported to the clinic for expensive hourly treatments.

The home therapy is safe, and can be assisted by a caregiver, and the patient efforts reduced from twice weekly therapy in clinics not equipped to treat the millions of patients to every other day therapy given at home, with a device less complicated that a CPAP device for sleep apnea.

WHY ISN'T HEALTHCARE MORE OPEN TO INNOVATION?

I spent most of my early career in the fast paced, competitive world of information technology, and was involved from before the IBM PC first launched in 1981. I got involved in healthcare in 1999, when I was fortunate to meet and begin working with Wilson Greatbatch, the inventor of the first successful implantable pacemaker, enabled by the low power requirements of transistors in the late 1950's. Wilson licensed his invention to a small company in Minneapolis, called Medtronic, went on their board, and the rest is history.
*http://www.electrohealing.com/about/wilson-greatbatch-memorial/greatbatch-articles/)

Having worked in both the fast paced IT and handheld computer industry, and the slow paced medical device industry, it is clear why the first moves fast and the latter quite slowly. One is competitive, the other feigns being competitive.

There are impediments at every stage along the way. Both in terms of approvals, perception and reputation.

What will help move this technology is awareness, by patients, physicians, clinicians, funders, hospital administrators, associations funding research, and the media. I have told you my story, and what I have learned.

Let's start a discussion and alert scientists and clinicians about the potential. That increases the chances someone will learn of it, and take an action to stop the pandemic.

I was lucky. I hope that the information in this book can help the many others suffering from dementia, whether Alzheimer's, TBI or other forms.

Please tell your friends and associates about it, and, if you want to help me continue the quest to get the technology recognized and adopted, you may wish to make a contribution to my gofundme project https://www.gofundme.com/stop-Alzheimer-s, or to the Quietmind Foundation (quietmindfdn.org),

Therein lies the cause of needless suffering of forty million human beings on this planet. Rich or poor, well connected or not.

ADDITIONAL INSIGHTS ON THE MECHANISM OF ACTION

It is not clear what the precise action is that causes photobiomodulation to achieve the treatment of Alzheimer's. Michael Hamblin's video and papers give a great overview of the possibilities.

http://photobiology.info/Hamblin.html

However, a breakthrough in understanding is coming as a result of the discoveries of Anirban Bandyopadhyay in Japan. He gave a presentation of how his discoveries may help explain how both light and ultrasound may both have beneficial effects on human health. I very much urge everyone to view this amazing video:

Anirban Bandyopadhyay- Where does music exist? - YouTube Video for anirban music microtubule▶ 12:52

https://www.youtube.com/watch?v=N5_fhIEmJI8

Discovery of Quantum Vibrations in "Microtubules" Inside Brain
- Elsevier https://www.elsevier.com/.../discovery-of-quantum-vibrations-in-microtubules... Elsevier
Jan 16, 2014 - Discovery of Quantum Vibrations in "Microtubules" Inside Brain Neurons ... brain neurons by the research group led by Anirban Bandyopadhyay, PhD, ... music, but unlike Western music which is harmonic," Hameroff explains.
Welcome to Anirban Bandyopadhyay Laboratory

www.anirbanlab.co.nr/

MAINTAINING MENTAL ACUITY

A study recently published shows how much keeping your mind active can help deter dementia. Here is a link to report covering that study:

http://www.latimes.com/science/sciencenow/la-sci-sn-brain-training-dementia-20160724-snap-story.html

Science Now
Discoveries from the world of science and medicine
Science Science Now

Brain training may forestall dementia onset for years, new study says
dementia computer training
Computerized braining training can hold off cognitive decline and dementia, new re-

search suggests.
(Carlos Chavez / Los Angeles Times)
Melissa Healy
If you're intent on keeping dementia at bay, new research suggests you'll need more than crossword puzzles, aerobic exercise and an active social life. In a study released Sunday, researchers found that older adults who did exercises to shore up the speed at which they processed visual information could cut by nearly half their likelihood of cognitive decline or dementia over a 10-year period.

OVERALL RECOMMENDATIONS

While I recommend you consult with a physician, I also recommend that you find a well read, open minded, non-arrogant one, if you can. I use several physicians, traditional, and alternative. Some take insurance, others do not. I make it clear to my physicians that I do not want my medical care to be based on allowable billing codes, but to keep these in mind and make me aware, as you are providing your most informed suggestions.

o diet and nutrition as indicated.

o neurofeedback improves attitude, mood and executive decision making.

o Near infrared light improves many bodily and cell functions, as explained in this book Get a device and use it. The increase in energy through ATP stimulation is very well indicated amongst those who study the literature.

o Other energy sources, TMS (transcranial magnetic stimulation), PEMF (pulsed electromagnetic stimulation), millimeter wave, and ultrasound (transcranial ultrasound or TUS), each have beneficial effects on our biological systems. These are just being understood and appreciated by the advanced guard of innovators in medicine. I believe they represent the next revolution in medicine.

o subscribe to alternative medical newsletters, but take things with some skepticism. Many things that offer a small benefit are marketed as if they might make difference in survival. They may not.

o I use a regular, insurance covered physician, and an alternative medicine MD and published physician who believes in anti-aging and longevity (Terry Grossman, MD, in Denver, CO) who works outside the limits of insurance coverage. He diagnosed my arteriosclerosis in 2002, and helped me reverse it in two years of therapy not covered by insurance, which I was able to get locally. Dr. Grossman is a member of the Association for the Advancement of Anti-Aging Medicine, which you can visit at A4M.org. They offer a free newsletter.

o What is not offered by modern medicine is tragically inefficient, Later in this book I list some of the causes for these inefficiencies. Most in healthcare hope to deliver innovations and enhancements. The system needs some changes.

DIET AND NUTRITION

It has become exceedingly clear that there is a direct connection between diet, nutrition, and health.

The ketogenic diet has been very well studied and is an excellent diet to help with Alzheimer's, TBI, cancer, and fighting and preventing other disease.

Here is a link to a site tracking all things Keto:
http://keto-everything.tumblr.com/

and a trailer for a movie about issues in the American diet:
http://keto-everything.tumblr.com/post/82871172554/fed-up-movie

My personal take is all people should engage in a combination of the following, whether as a preventative, or to fight a diagnosed condition.

Each of us, by understanding these, can contribute to needed change.

o A company took patents licensed from the University of South Florida (USF) and developed a daily drink that provides the essential food that the ketogenic diet requires (you have to consume the food for the diet to work). They improved the science and the process, and take the hassle out of following this diet, which studies indicate has the potential to correct the detriments of the non-healthy American diet. You can get their product at this web-site:
www.kegenix.com

o This preview for an excellent movie on diet is very much every American watching:
http://keto-everything.tumblr.com/post/82871172554/fed-up-movie

A series of excellent publications is available University Health News (UHN) at the link below. I have copied some of the material to show you the depth and breadth. By visiting the site you can download a book on Alzheimer's you may find very helpful.

Here is a very useful link from University Health News:

http://universityhealthnews.com/daily/memory/ketogenic-diet-shows-promising-results-for-all-dementia-stages/

Ketogenic Diet Shows Promising Results for All Dementia Stages

BY UHN STAFF • OCT 28, 2015
READ COMMENTS (5)

We all know that a poor diet causes weight gain, heart disease and diabetes. But did you know that your brain can be affected by your diet just as much as your waistline can? Fortunately, as a healthy diet can help you shed unwanted pounds, it can also prevent unwanted memory loss. By "feeding" your brain the nutrients it needs, you can actually improve your memory and thwart the development of dementia, including Alzheimer's.

Studies show a ketogenic diet can slow and even reverse symptoms of memory loss and cognitive impairment throughout all the dementia stages.

TREATMENT FOR DEPRESSION

http://www.fisherwallace.com/

http://www.brainsway.com/us/patients-portal

https://neurostar.com/?utm_source=bing&utm_medium=cpc&utm_campaign=Patient_Neurostar_Magnetic%20Stimulation&utm_term=magnet%20treatment%20for%20depression&utm_content=Neurostar_Magnetic%20Stimulation_Broad

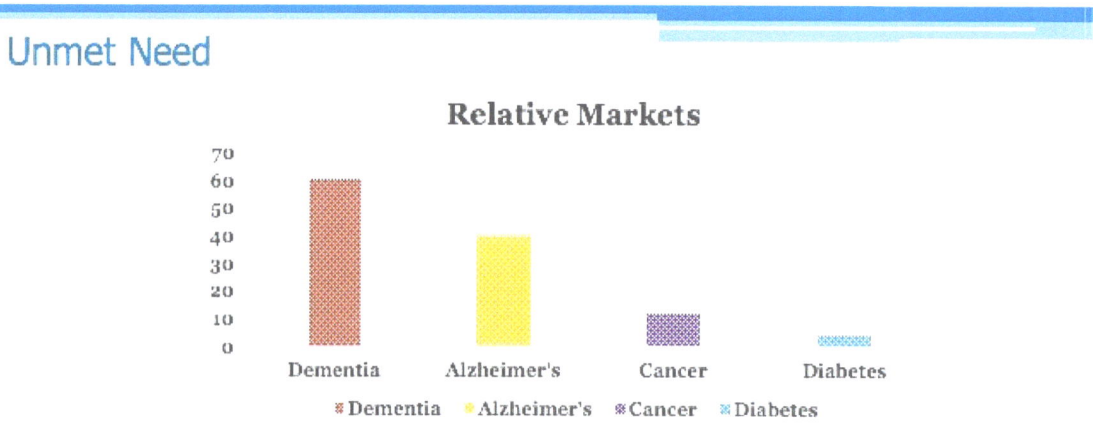

source:Dallas Hack, MD MPH in a presentation to scientists in 2016

Indications in laboratory experiments with human patients have shown that these technologies may also help patients with:

tinnitus, dementia, TBI, PTSD, ADHD

The discovery can be called Nanowaves.

Breakthrough Discovery:

Nanowaves^{tm}

- We all know that light can be both a wave and a particle.

- However, we did not realize that nanowaves can impact human cells and induce healing outcomes, non-invasively, and transcranially.

- No particles required! No brain barrier to penetrate. No cutting, drilling, infusing. No sepsis.

- As were minimally-invasive technologies when first brought to the clinic: balloon angioplasty, laparoscopy, valves, stents, et al.

It remains a serious socio-economic problem that the NIH and the Alzheimer's Association do not pursue these potential therapies. And the large device companies do not. So, who has the concern of the 5 million Alzheimer's patients in their sights? (source: Dallas Hack, MD):

Problem

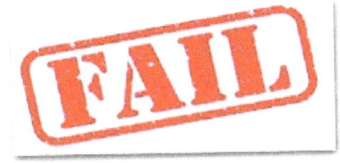

Current Alzheimer's Disease Treatment Leads to Poor Outcomes

Ineffective Symptom Management
Radical Mental and Physical Decline
Loved ones remembered in debilitated state
   - affects all demographics
Extremely High Costs (Over $600 billion)

Please contribute to our efforts, and please tell your friends, neighbors, co-works and congressional representatives that the healthcare industry is not taking advantage of the needs of its citizens.

Also, give your physician a copy of this book. And, if you have a loved one in need of therapy, contact any of the following to find about IRB approved clinical trials that may be available near you.

The Quietmind Foundation (www.quietmiwww.quietmindfdnndfdn,com)

Lumineu, Inc. (www.lumineu.com) and its affiliate: NooThera.com

STRATEGY TO CHANGE MEDICINE

Although medicine is slow to, it does eventually innovate.

Several things are essential to change.

o   Data - which we have and are growing
o   Money - which we are now raising
o   Management - which we have, from industry, defense and academia.
o   Intellectual Property - this may have been the holdback, since light therapy is now approaching twenty years and many of the early patents have expired. There are pending and issued patents that Lumineu has been rolling up.

Lumineu, a company formed by scientists, physicians, clinicians, patent attorneys, and entrepreneurs, has decided to make the first system with both light therapy and neurofeedback, combined, and make it portable for use in home, assisted living or clinic, and affordable. It will be automated so, once the physician provides a prescription for use, it is easier to use than a CPAC machine for sleep therapy.

It is the first device to be fully automated for home use, to eliminate twice weekly trips to the therapist, and expensive hourly visits. The patient gets an initial QEEG brain scan from the physician and therapist, and a home prescription is provided into the safe, automated home or bedside unit that can be used 2-3 times weekly, by the patient or caregiver, and monitored remotely by the therapists, who advises the physician.

This automated innovation should lower the cost of therapy, per patient, from $50,000 per year, to under $10,000, and reduce trips to the therapist from 100 per year, to approximately four.

Full details on this company can be found at this site: https://app.box.com/s/77b-szm2x57zm1ukwsdjitygcqnxxuti5

The company's web site is lumineu.com. An affiliate site, NooThera.com also has useful technical data.

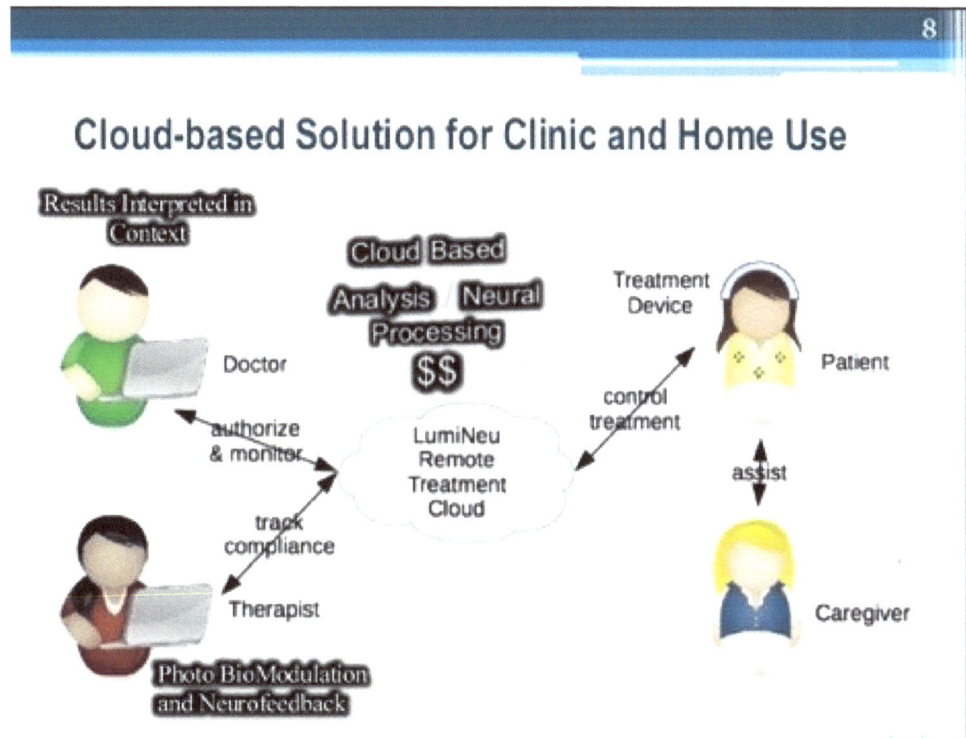

For full disclosure, I am one of the inventors on the patents, and I am an investor and co-founder in Lumineu.

The strategy deployed by Lumineu includes designing the proprietary automated home therapy system, using what has been covered in patent applications and additional issued IP, and be the first to market,. They will deploy telemedicine for individualized therapy at affordable low cost systems with more sophisticated systems in the clinic.

These device can incorporate other technologies, including healing energy, pain management, integration with imaging devices, and integration with the therapist and patient, at home.

These patents are pioneering, and delineate entirely new therapy and devices enabling the next revolution in medicine.

Here a few selected drawings from the first two patents and foreign equivalents.

This embodiment describes how a multi-frequency laser can send healing energy to any square-centimeter on a patient's head, to up or down regulated desired outcomes on a patient in a clinic. This can allow, as an example, treating one area of the brain needing healing energy, without increasing mania in the patient, or uptake of pharmaceuticals, in other areas.

The use of multi-frequency therapy can be directed to other parts of the body. Scientific publications report that even opioids can be induced in the

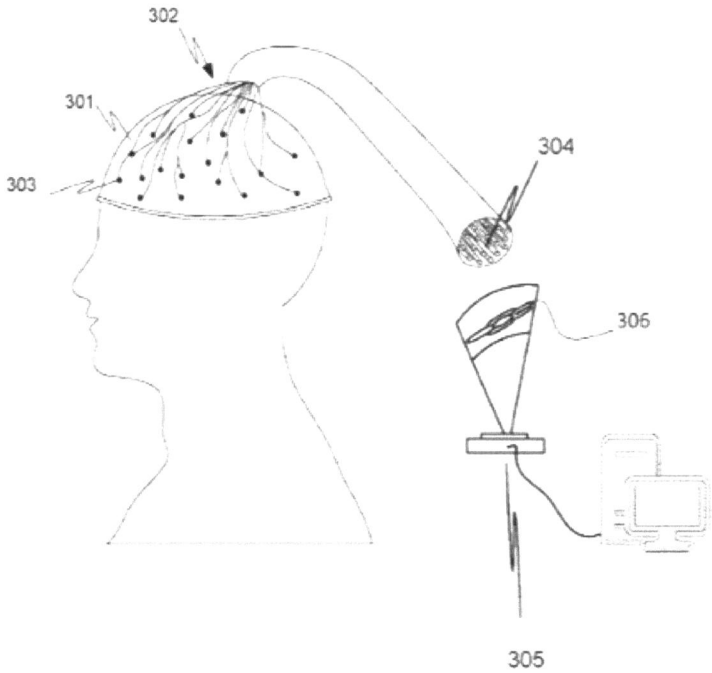

FIG. 3

DOCKET NUMBER: NTL0001NP

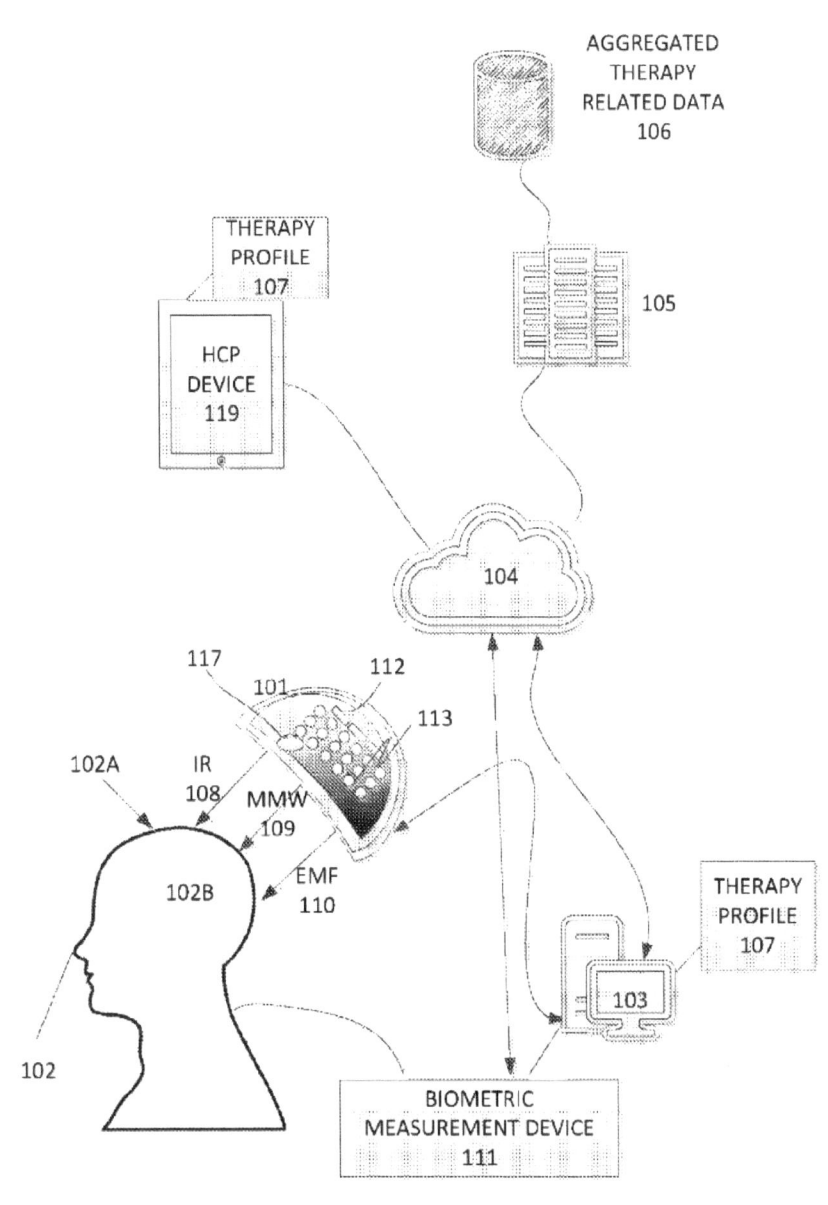

FIG. 1

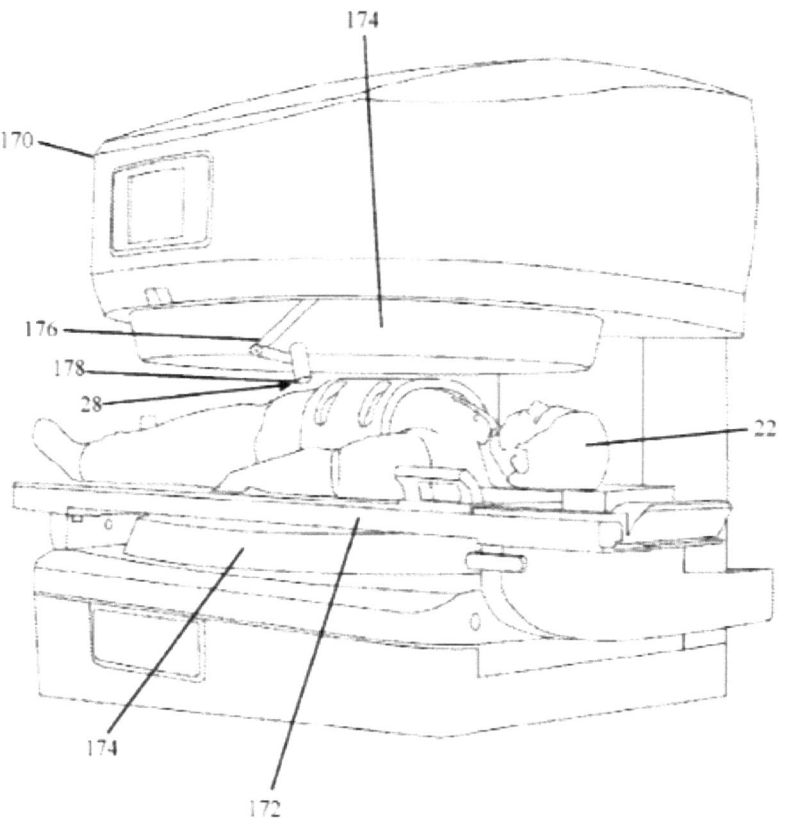

170

174

176

178

28

22

174

172

Fig. 17

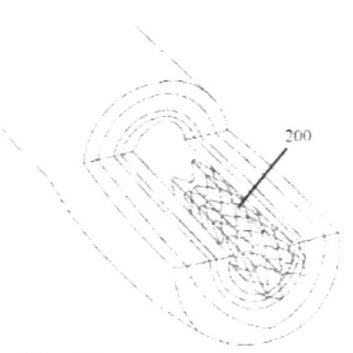

Fig. 20

Docket Number: NTL0002NP

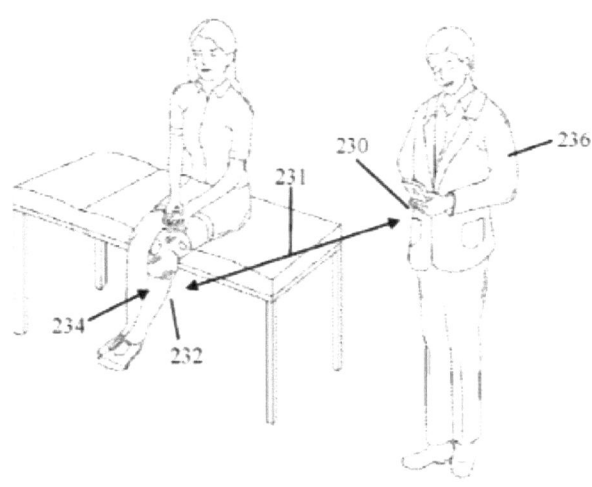

Fig. 23

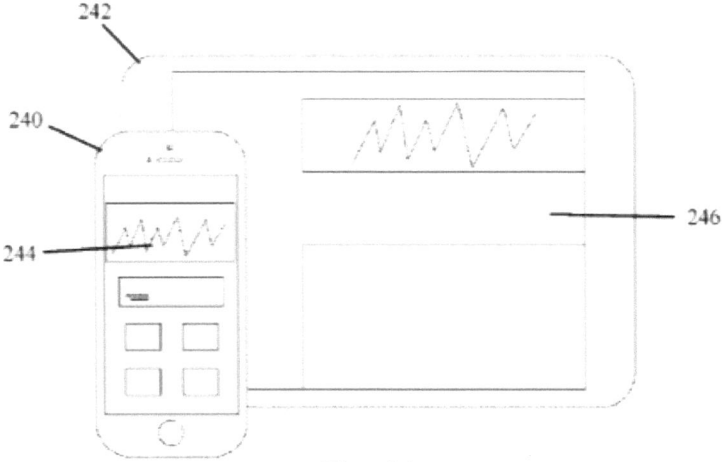

Fig. 24

Docket Number: NTL0002NP

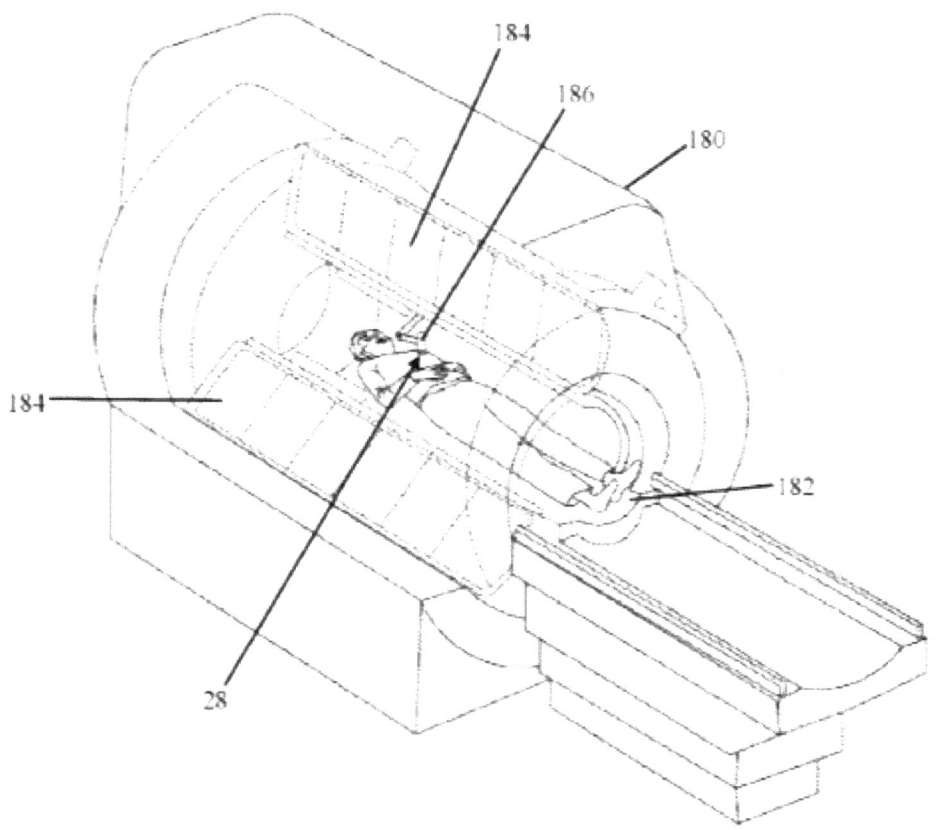

184
186
180
184
182
28

Fig. 18

47

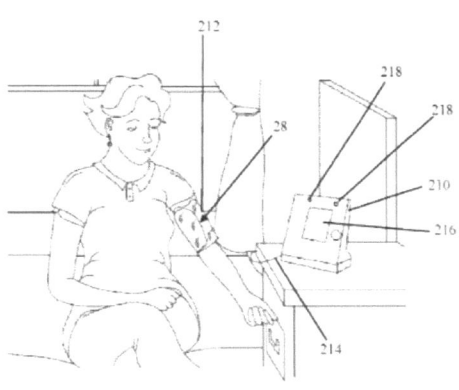

Fig. 21

Here is a link to the omnibus patent filings (patent filings designed to birth many future patents and claims, over time):

Lumineu has acquired the **patent applications** of NooThera LLC, as well as licenses being acquired for other IP. Here are several pending patents applied for, which also have foreign equivalents on file:

https://app.box.com/files/0/f/7151373249/1/f_74251376662

These patents teach how several treatments can be combined into a device or method. Infrared light that can be enhanced with neurofeedback, nearly doubling the measurable cognitive effect of either, on their own.

Light therapy appears to stop degeneration, and neurofeedback improves cognition.

The patents cover many innovations, including how to combine multiple therapies into clinical systems, and how to automate home therapy, connected by telemedicine, to make the cost of care affordable.

The combination appears patentable over the prior art.

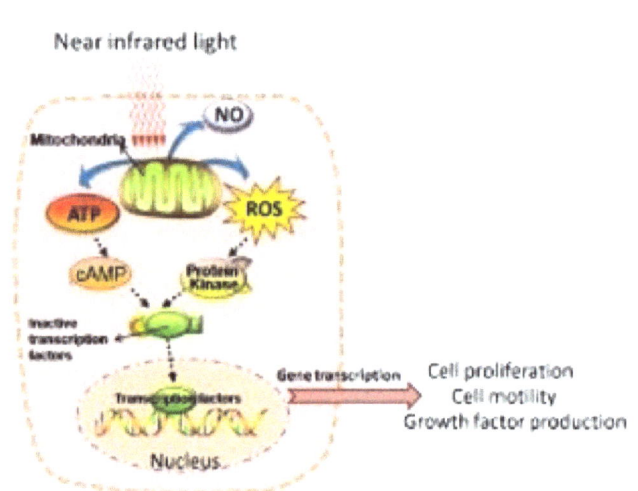

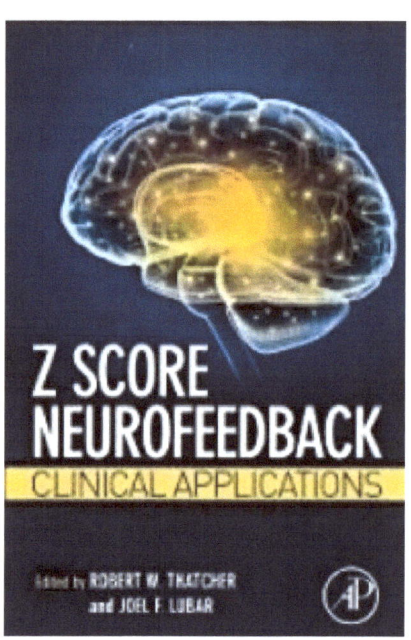

PUBLICATIONS ON THE USE OF LLLT OR PHOTOBIOMODULATION

Selection of PBM-Alzheimer's Articles

Low-Level Laser Therapy to the Bone Marrow Ameliorates Neurodegenerative Disease Progression in a Mouse Model of Alzheimer's Disease: A Minireview
Oron Amir and Oron Uri. Photomedicine and Laser Surgery. June 2016, ahead of print. doi:10.1089/pho. 2015.4072.
www.ncbi.nlm.nih.gov/pubmed/27294393

PBM Can Arrest Neuronal Death
Turning On Lights to Stop Neurodegeneration: The Potential of Near Infrared Light Therapy in Alzheimer's and Parkinson's Disease
Daniel M. Johnstone, Cécile Moro, Jonathan Stone, Alim-Louis Benabid, and John Mitrofanis,* Front Neurosci. 2015; 9: 5nk Luis, Rodríguez-Santana Elizabeth, Santana-Rodríguez Karin E., and Reyes Heberto. Photomedicine and Laser Surgery. March 2016, 34(3): 93-101. doi:10.1089/pho.2015.4015. www.ncbi.nlm.nih.gov/pubmed/26890728

Alzheimers Research

PBM Increases Cognitive Function

Low-level laser therapy ameliorates disease progression in a mouse model of Alzheimer's disease.
Farfara D, Tuby H, Trudler D, Doron-Mandel E, Maltz L, Vassar RJ, Frenkel D, Oron U. J Mol Neurosci. 2015 Feb; 55(2):430-6. doi: 10.1007/s12031-014-0354-z. Epub 2014 Jul 4.

PBM Increase BDNF

Low-level laser therapy promotes dendrite growth via upregulating brain-derived neurotrophic factor expression Chengbo Meng ; Zhiyong He and Da Xing, Proc. SPIE 9230, Twelfth International Conference on Photonics and Imaging in Biology and Medicine (PIBM 2014), 92301G (September 17, 2014); doi:10.1117/12.2068980; http:// dx.doi.org/10.1117/12.2068980proceedings.spiedigitallibrary.org/proceeding.aspx?articleid=1907067

PBM Reduces Tau Tangles and β-amyloid Plaques

Photobiomodulation with near infrared light mitigates Alzheimer's disease-related pathology in cerebral cortex – evidence from two transgenic mouse models. Sivaraman Purushothuman, Daniel M JohnstoneEmail author, Charith Nandasena, John Mitrofanis and Jonathan Stone. Alzheimer's Research & Therapy 20146:2 DOI: 10.1186/alzrt232 https://alzres.biomedcentral.com/articles/10.1186/alzrt232

PBM I

PBM Can Suppress Neuroinflammation Pre-conditioning with transcranial low-level light therapy reduces neuroinflammation and protects blood-brain barrier after focal cerebral ischemia in mice. Lee, Hae Ina | Park, Jung Hwab | Park, Min Youngb | Kim, Nam Gyunc | Park, Kyoung-Junc | Choi, Byung Taeb | Shin, Yong-IIa | Shin, Hwa Kyoung; Restorative Neurology and Neuroscience, vol. 34, no. 2, pp. 201-214, 2016 DOI: 10.3233/RNN-150559 content.iospress.com/articles/restorative-neurology-and-neuroscience/rnn150559
PBM Increases BDNF After TBI
Low-level laser therapy for traumatic brain injury in mice increases brain derived neurotrophic factor (BDNF) and synaptogenesis
Weijun Xuan, Tanupriya Agrawal, Liyi Huang, Gaurav K. Gupta and Michael R. Hamblin Journal of Biophotonics Volume 8, Issue 6, pages 502–511, June 2015 DOI: 10.1002/jbio.201400069 onlinelibrary.wiley.com/doi/10.1002/jbio.201400069/ abstract;jsessionid=9739CFEE73B256EFD1D1082A7F71C21A.f03t03

PBM Improves Mitochondrial Respiration
Mitochondrial respiration as a target for neuroprotection and cognitive enhancement.
Gonzalez-Lima F, Barksdale BR, Rojas JC. Biochem Pharmacol. 2014 Apr 15;88(4):584-93. doi: 10.1016/j.bcp.2013.11.010. Epub 2013 Dec 4.

NEUROFEEDBACK REFERENCES

LORETA Z Score Neurofeedback - EEG Acquistion and Analysis www.appliedneuroscience.com/LORETAZScoreNF.htm

Read Testimonials on EEG Neurofeedback - NeuroGuide by Applied ... www.appliedneuroscience.com/TestimonialNF.htm
Jun 12, 2016 - My guess is you have taken neurofeedback training to a "new level." ... I did several sessions of LORETA and surface Z score training the past ... 3-Dimensional LORETA Z Score Neurofeedback neurofeedback-loreta.com/

Neurofeedback. Operant conditioning of the electrical activity of the brain using Low Resolution Brain Electromagnetic Tomography (LORETA).
Neurofeedback and EEG Biofeedback Treatment www.thebrainperformancecenter.com/our-programs/neurofeedback/

With Z score training you may be training eight to ten metrics, and with LORETA Z score you may train hundreds of metrics at the same time. You can alter how ...
Z-score LORETA Neurofeedback as a Potential Therapy for Patients ... https://sciforschenonline.org/journals/neurology/NOA-1-101.php
Citation: Koberda JL and Frey LC (2015) Z-score LORETA Neurofeedback as a Potential Therapy for

Patients with Seizures and Refractory Epilepsy. Neurol ... 3-Dimensional LORETA Z Score Neurofeedback for ... - bio-medical.com
bio-medical.com/.../neuroguide-add-on-nf2-3-dimensional-loreta-z-score- neurofeedb...
19 channel neurofeedback trains the brain using z-scores. This can be thought of as

... LORETA neurofeedback is based on the work of Robert Thatcher, PhD. Browsing Store - 19Ch 3-D
LORETA Z-Score NFT - BrainMaster store.brainmaster.com/browse.cfm/4,313.html

19 channel 3-Dimensional LORETA Z-Score Neurofeedback for NeuroGuide Deluxe Z-Score biofeedback of Brodmann areas in the brain. "Hubs", "Modules" ...
Live Z-Score Training | BrainMaster Neurofeedback www.brainmaster.com/content-sub/live-z-score-
training/

Deep Brain Neurofeedback | Electromagnetic Tomography (LoRETA ... www.brainworksneurothera-
py.com › methods

It is uniquely capable of neurofeedback directly on deep brain areas and functions; as well as Hag-
mann's Hubs, Modules, and Default Mode Networks. The symptom checklist is combined with LORE-
TA Z scores measured during a QEEG analysis to aid in linking patient's symptoms to functional spe-
cialisation in the brain.

NeuroGuide Add-on NF2. Combines surface EEG LORETA Z scores measured during a QEEG analysis
to further aid in the development of a neurofeedback ... 19 Channel Neurofeedback - Scottsdale Neurofeedback Institute, AZ scottsdaleneurofeedback.com/services/19-channel-neurofeedback/

www.appliedneuroscience.com

SELECTION OF LIGHT THERAPY DEVICES THAT ARE WITHIN THE SAME RANGE OF SUCCESSFUL CLINICAL TRIALS STUDIES

VIELIGHT (www.vielight.com)

Vielight makes a device designed to combine light therapy at 810 nanometers, using LED's, laser diodes, or actually low power lasers, that radiate a key part of the brain where Alzheimer's and TBI are often beginning, and in addition to stabilizing degeneration, they also help induce the "plasticity," as it is now called, which is the ability of the brain to reform wiring and functionality. This prepares the brain for the essential neurofeedback therapy, pioneered by Dr. Marvin Berman of the Quietmind Foundation (quietmindfdn.org). It is not known if it generates enough light to penetrate the cranium to the cortex of the brain to treat Alzheimer's.

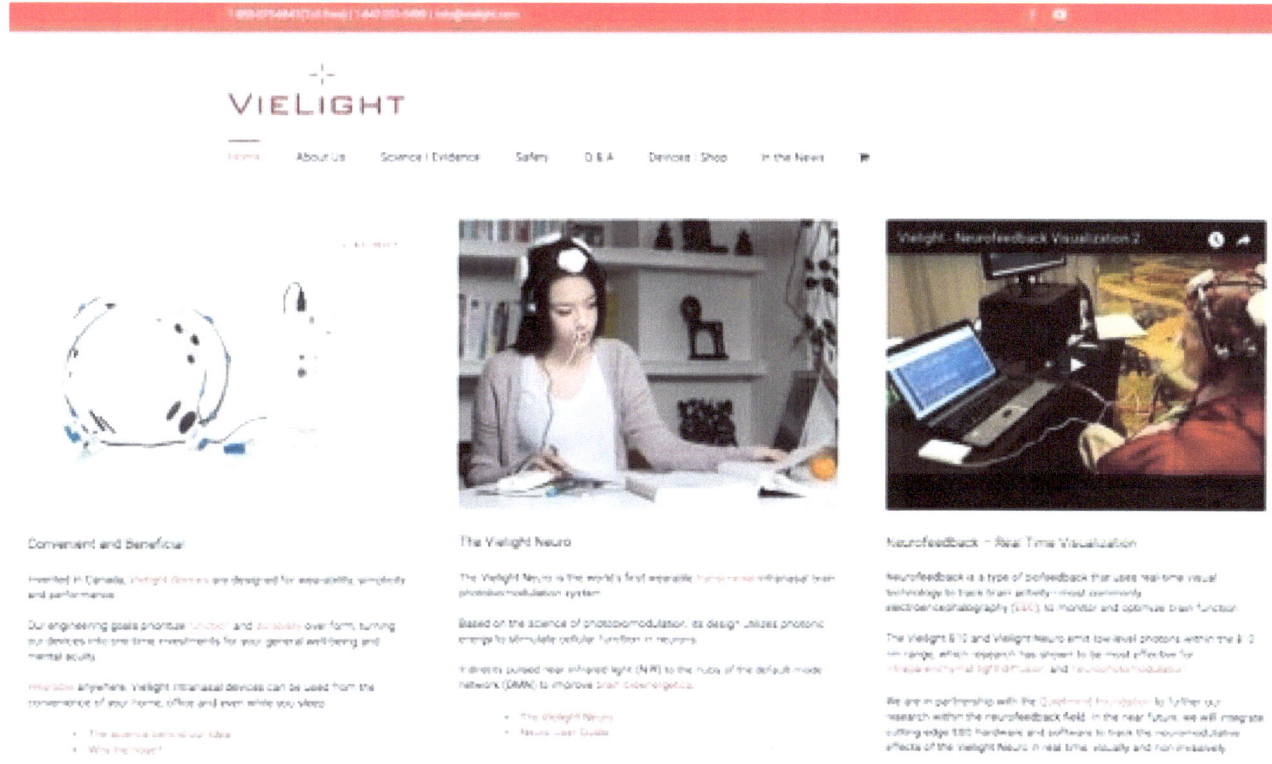

In addition to the head worn unit, a device that puts infrared into your nose has the benefits of shining on an area where there is significant exposure to the blood, as well as penetration into the brain. Founder and CEO Lew Lim, Ph.D. has been leading the effort to get awareness and devices onto the market for the general public, without medical indication, while doing some of the leading research in conjunction with Harvard's Wellman Research Center, and the Quiet-mind Foundation:

THE LEDMAN (THELEDMAN.com)

This is an inexpensive, quite effective, affordable device that is available in 660, 850, or a combination of the two frequencies. Additionally, on request, for a small additional fee, they will make available a custom 830 nanometer version. Our studies of the literature indicate that 830 is the best frequency to get for brain stimulation and penetration, and may also be very helpful for pain relief of the back, and neck. We recommend the custom 830 over the dual 660/850, for minimal dosing time and optimal performance.

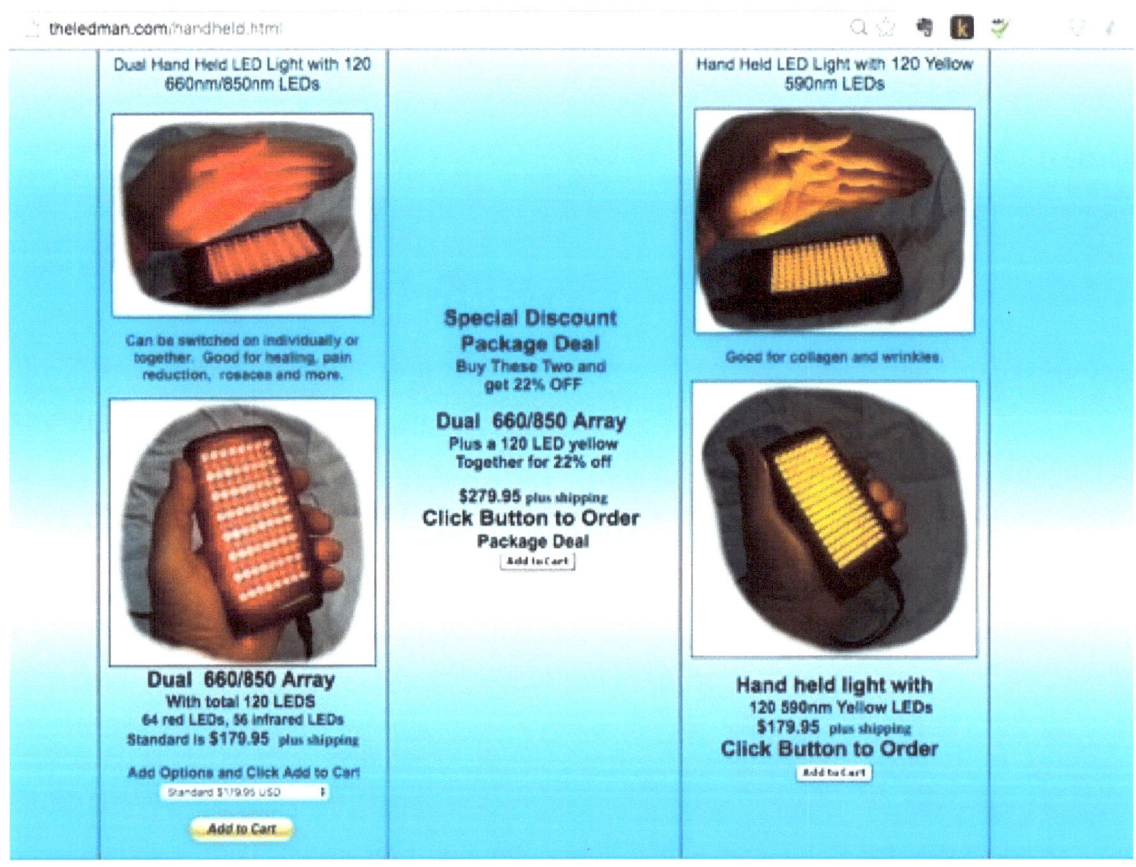

LITE CURE
www.litecure.com

One of the industry leaders, you can use Litecure's site to find a therapist near you with their powerful equipment, request a demonstration, or order a device. Physicians, chiropractors and clinics may wish to explore their devices, designed for long term active use in the clinic or sports medicine practice.

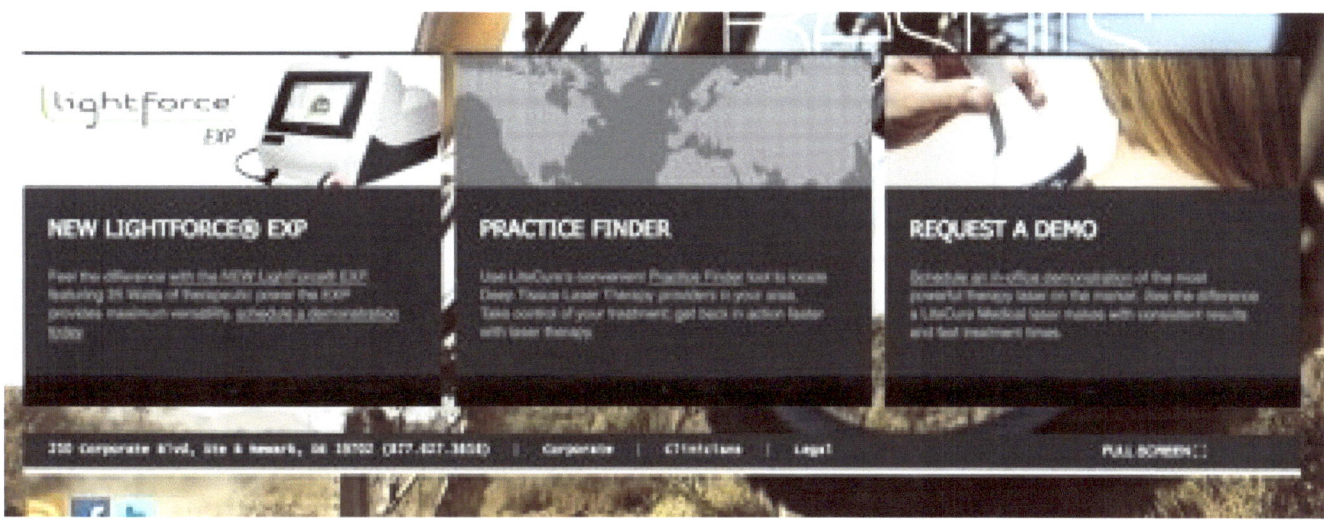

THOR LASER (www.thorlaser.com)

Another of the industrial and research leaders in the industry. Based in the UK, they market worldwide to clinics, spas, and gyms.

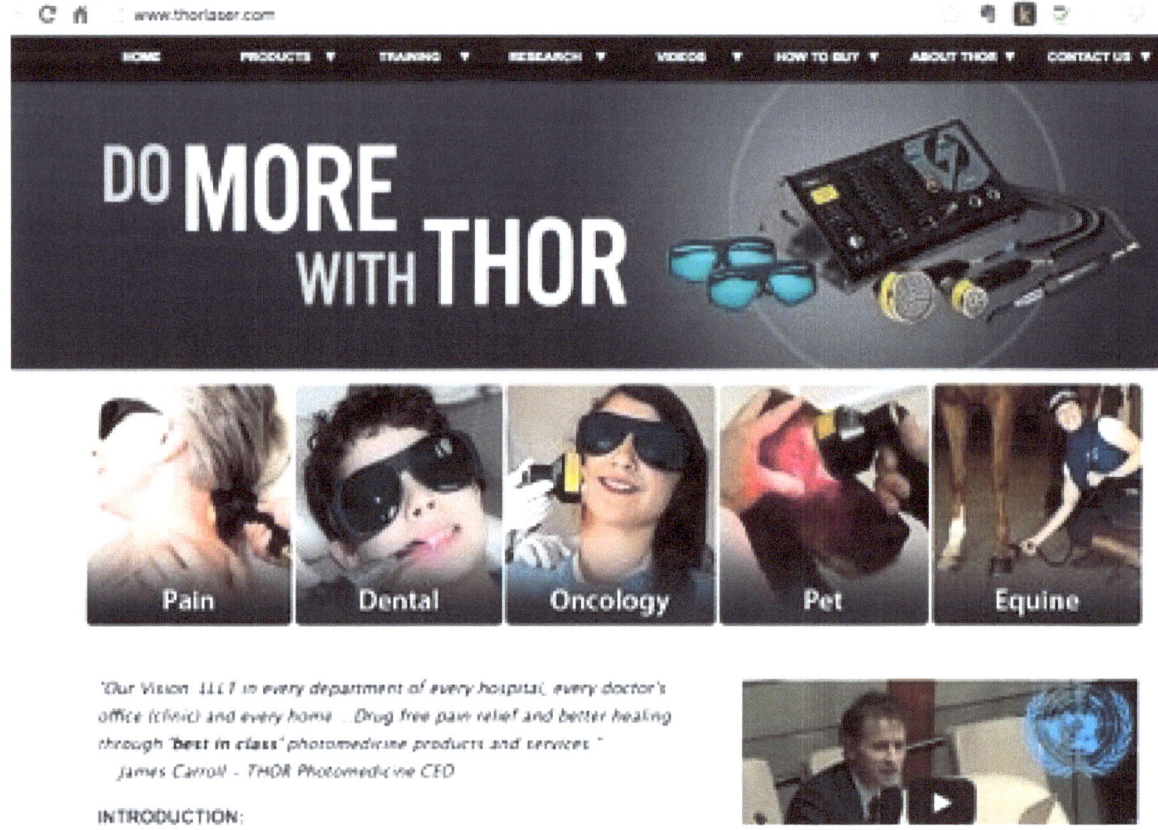

"Our Vision 1117 in every department of every hospital, every doctor's office (clinic) and every home ... Drug free pain relief and better healing through 'best in class' photomedicine products and services."
James Carroll - THOR Photomedicine CEO

INTRODUCTION:

THE BRAIN BUFFER

This device, called the Brain Buffer, is to be on the market end of 2016, competes with the $1,000 plus units, with the benefit of a very high light energy output in the 830 nanometer range, allowing for much shorter dosing times. It features a curved shape to allow fitting more closely to the head's curved shape, to more of the LED lights touch the cranium.

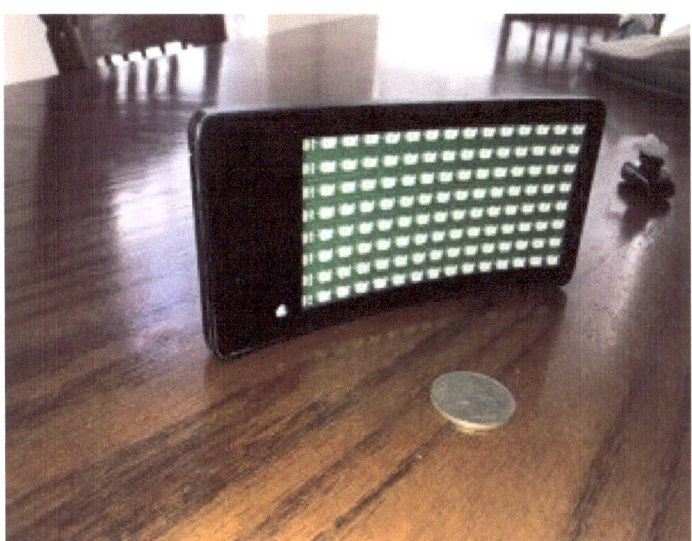

We received this early prototype and were quite impressed with the compact size, portability and design. Write for more information in the second half of 2016, when they will have information on where to buy it (info@electrohealiing.com).

It provides the non-invasive light energy for the types of applications described here. It's power output and design using 120 of the newer, high power LED's, with greater penetration allow for 6-10 minute dosing, versus most others at 20 minutes. It has the wattage output approaching much more expensive devices, and works in the desired low 800 nanometer near infrared range.

Patients and their physicians, reading the evidence in this book and the scientific literature, have to make a choice as to what to do when the medical device industry is not servicing the many soldiers suffering from TBI or the many people suffering from the horrific tragedy of Alzheimer's.

My hope is that some physicians and patients will undertake studies under the appropriate legal auspices, and others will alert their congressional representatives, foundation representatives, an hospital administrators to get the word out, so that the industry standing between scientists and the clinics acts, or cedes its market dominance to more competitive and innovative organizations.

EQUINE LASERS

One of the most remarkable things you will discover as you investigate cold lasers for low level light therapy (LLLT, aka PBM), is the range in cost, frequency, power and features.

Even more remarkable is how well these devices are known and used by dentists, and also in sports medicine clinics, chiropractic offices, and horse doctors. Devices that can regenerate gums in humans, could also be restoring heart tissue, kidneys, livers, and other tissue and organs, if it were not for the arrogant bias7575 that permeates much of allopathic medicine. Unfortunately, the pure bias and bigotry has suppressed the pioneering medical evidence that has permeated the research clinic for the past twenty years, and bypassed most of modern medicine.

These suppliers are a viable alternative to purchase both LED devices or lasers.

The following table includes lasers that sell on ColdLasers.Org as well as other popular lasers.

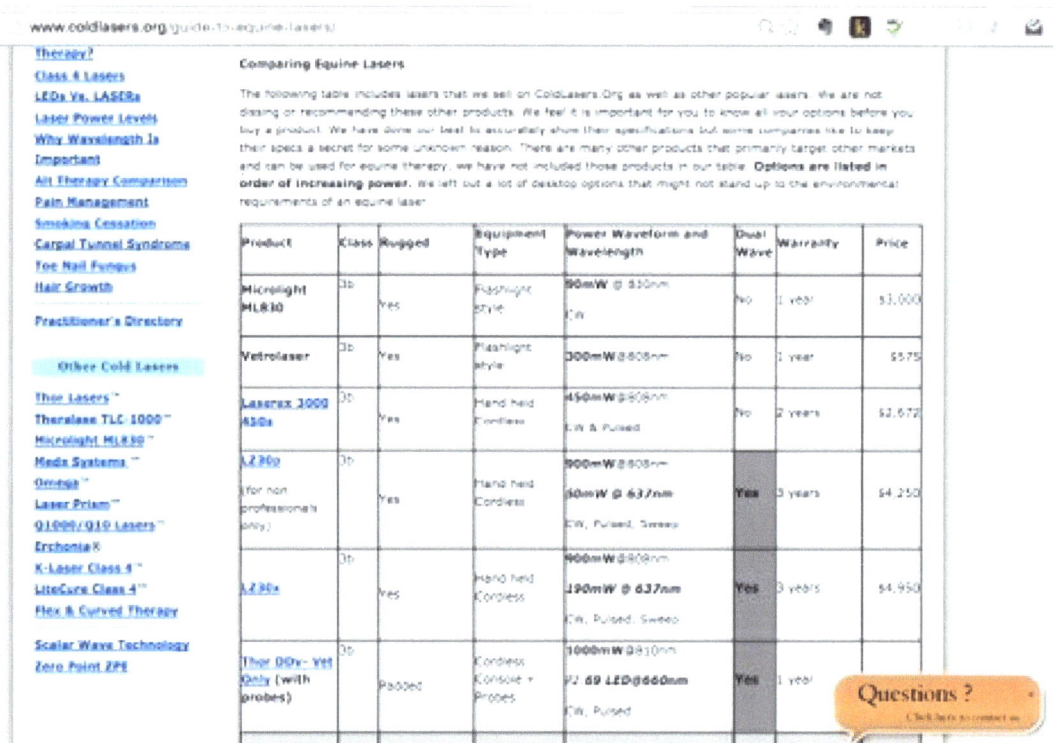

I particularly like the Vetrolaser at 808 nanometers, and some places offer a two frequency device, for as low as $450!

VETROLASER

Therapeutic Lasers You Can Afford
Infrared Laser Packages From $575.00 Plus $15.00 Shipping.
30 Day Money Back Guarantee. Two Year Product Guarantee.

Order Soon And Get A Bonus Single Diode Acupuncture Laser

Sold For Animal Use Only

1-800-742-8433 info@vetrolaser.com
Dr. Daniel Kamen, D.C. will personally answer the phone and all of your questions.

Home Page

Shop Online

Video Demo

FAQ

Testimonials

Adjusting Clips And More

Cold Laser Links

More Laser Info

Free Horse Chiro WkBook

Horse Chiro Seminar

1-800-742-8433 or 708-744-6325 Email us here:
This is the same cold laser used by thousands of veterinarians worldwide.

Quickly Treat Wounds, Joints, Bowed Tendons, Muscles, And Pain

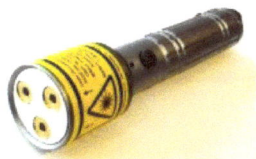 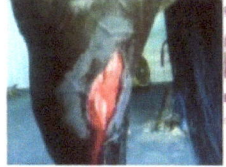 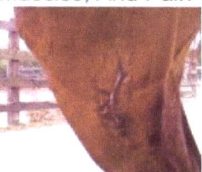

Vetrolaser 808nm/300mW   Horse Wound Before And Eight Weeks After Using The Vetrolaser*

Veterinarians Use Our Lasers To Treat Pain Associated With Canine Hip Dysplasia And ACL Tears.

Treat Sores On Dogs Commonly Found On Their Paws (Pads) And Legs.

Same Day Shipping. Ships By USPS Priority Mail

Click On Our Online Store For Discounts When You Buy Two Laser Packages

Vetrolaser Video Demo: http://www.youtube.com/watch?v=IYTTvPo3j5Y

Note: When we mail your laser package by USPS priority mail, we send it requiring a signature, assuring the customer receives their purchase. Please let us know in advance if you prefer not to sign for it.

Why Pay Thousands? "Ours Does Exactly What Theirs Does For A Fraction Of The Price."

Veterinarian Recommended

"I purchased my Vetrolaser weeks ago, and began utilizing it immediately on my canine and feline patients. Not only have I noticed tremendous decrease in post-operative inflammation, but my clients are very happy I am including this as a treatment modality. Since there are many posts about how well the unit works, I will not overkill the issue. The one thing I notice that appears to not be mentioned is the financial benefit. The unit has paid for itself within two weeks, making this purchase a no-brainer. Thanks again Dr. Kamen."

G. Roiland, DVM

"If you still have your heart set on spending $5,000.00 for a real infrared cold laser, then buy 10 of ours." Ours are *real* lasers, <u>NOT</u> LED's.
Did you know that some people spend over $12,000.00 for a 635nm/5mW red laser? Did you also know that you get a FREE single diode red laser with those specifications when you buy the Vetrolaser?

Our Cold Laser Packages

The **$575.00** package (plus $15.00 shipping)

58

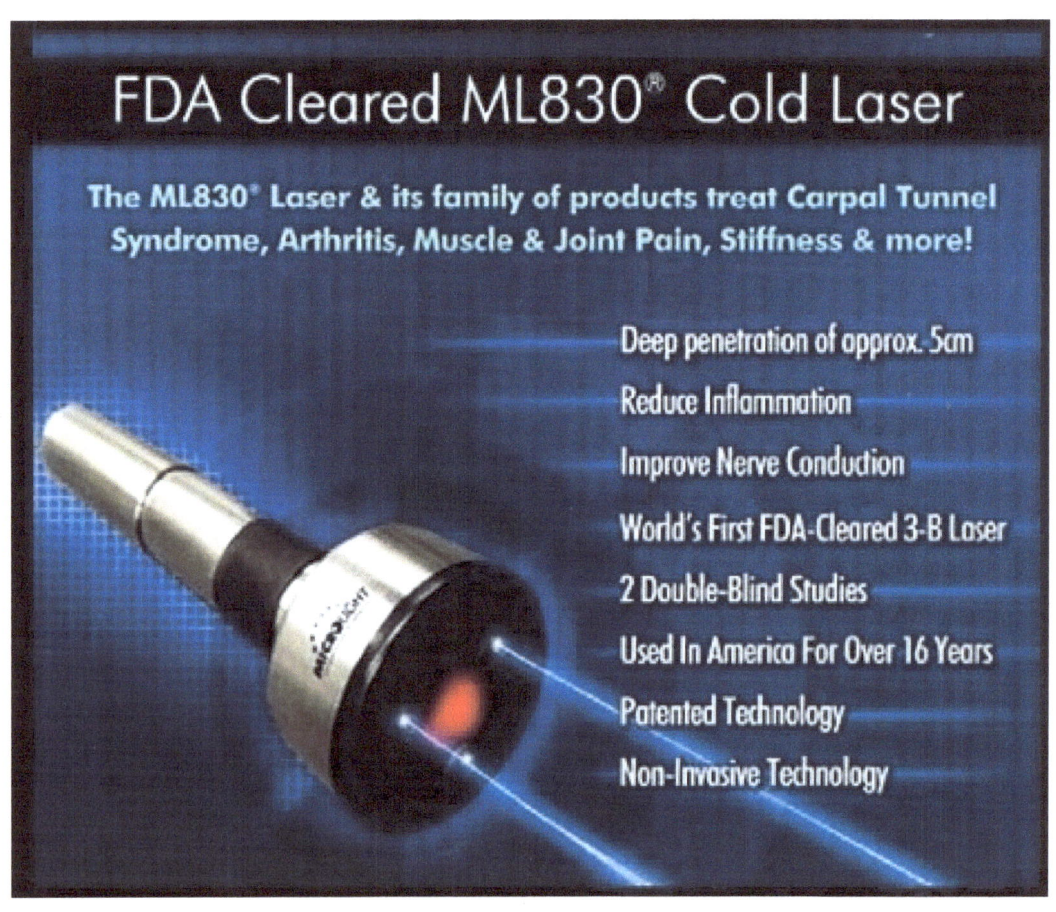

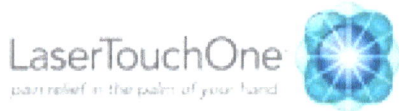
LaserTouchOne
pain relief in the palm of your hand

ABOUT US   CUSTOMER SERVICE   FIND A DEALER   CONTACT

HOME   ERASE PAIN   HOW IT WORKS   STUDIES & SUCCESS   BUY NOW

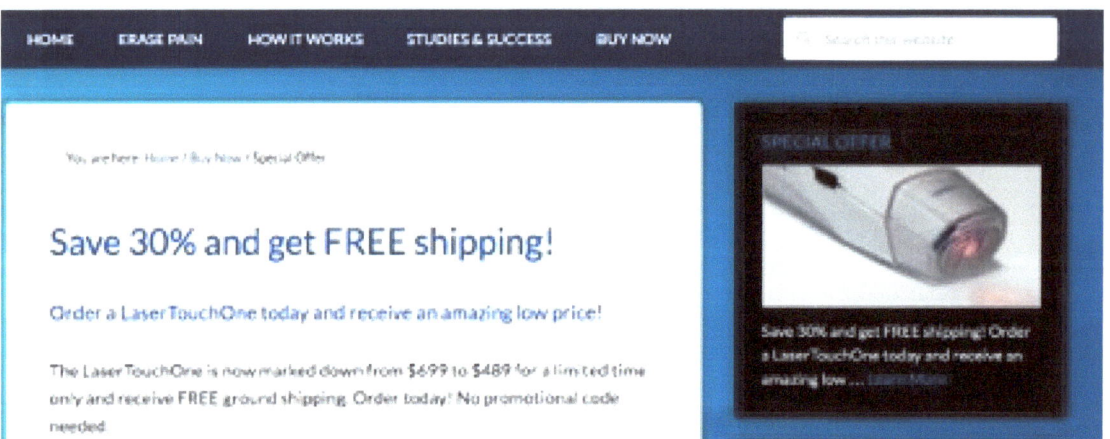

You are here: Home / Buy Now / Special Offer

Save 30% and get FREE shipping!

Order a LaserTouchOne today and receive an amazing low price!

The LaserTouchOne is now marked down from $699 to $489 for a limited time only and receive FREE ground shipping. Order today! No promotional code needed.

SPECIAL OFFER

Save 30% and get FREE shipping! Order a LaserTouchOne today and receive an amazing low ... Learn More

LaserTouchOne™ Specifications

Laser	
LASER Type	Laser Diode
Wavelength	670nm +/- 10nm
Power	1.2mW
Transcutaneous Electrical Nerve Stimulation	
Waveform shape	Biased, rectangular
Maximum output voltage	18 V @ 500 ohm load
	150 V @ 10K ohm load
Maximum output current	90 mA peak at 500 ohm load
Pulse width	6 – 80 μm.
Frequency	65 Hz +/- 10%
Pulse period	22 mS
Maximum current density	0.25 mA/cm2 average @ 500 ohms
Maximum power density	0.0011 W/cm2 average @ 500 ohms
Maximum charge per pulse	16 μJ @ 500 ohms or 2.4 μC @ 500 ohms
Power	
Rechargeable Battery	Lithium Ion

About The Developer

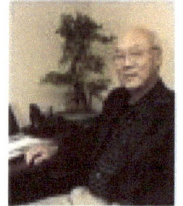

For Dr. Okky Oei, the quest for finding solutions for both chronic and acute pain started with his own back injury years ago. Dr. Oei quickly realized that most of the medications used to treat pain were accompanied by significant side effects that were difficult to tolerate. His personal need to relieve his own pain without experiencing the debilitating effects of heavy medications prompted him to find scientific, evidence-based, non-medicinal, non-invasive treatment. It was Dr. Oei's vision that pain relief could (and should) be achieved by addressing the source of pain rather than simply treating symptoms.

Okky Oei, M.D.

Dr. Oei began his pain relief practice quest and utilized many traditional and complementary treatments such as trigger point injections, acupuncture and myofascial release techniques. He then studied and used micro current electrical stimulation to achieve significant pain relief results for his patients. His next steps in research and testing involved low level laser therapy (LLLT), a treatment modality that was being used worldwide but still in its infancy in the US.

61

CELASERS
WWW.CELASERS.COM

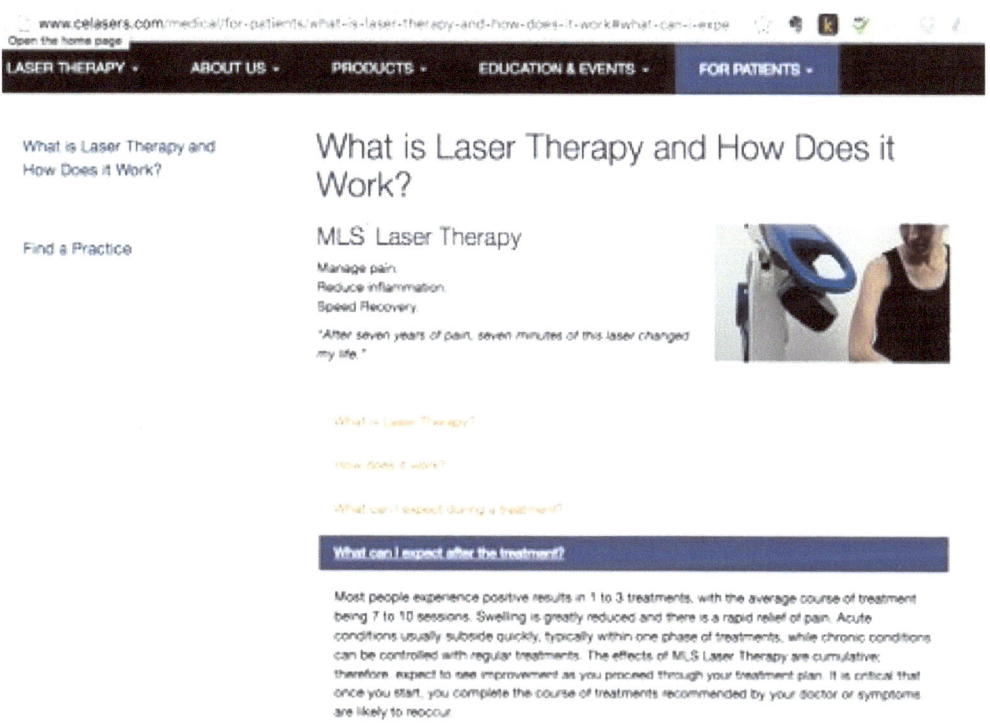

M6 – Robotic MLS Therapy Laser

The M6 therapy laser is a robotized multi-target device designed to treat patients suffering pathologies affecting a wide area, and to perform automatic applications. The distinctive feature of the M6 is the innovative multi-target functioning. Thanks to the features of the exclusive MLS multi-diodic optical group, a wide area is treated instantaneously helping to produce an immediate response of the treated tissues. The results are better and faster than with the scanning modality of traditional laser therapy products.

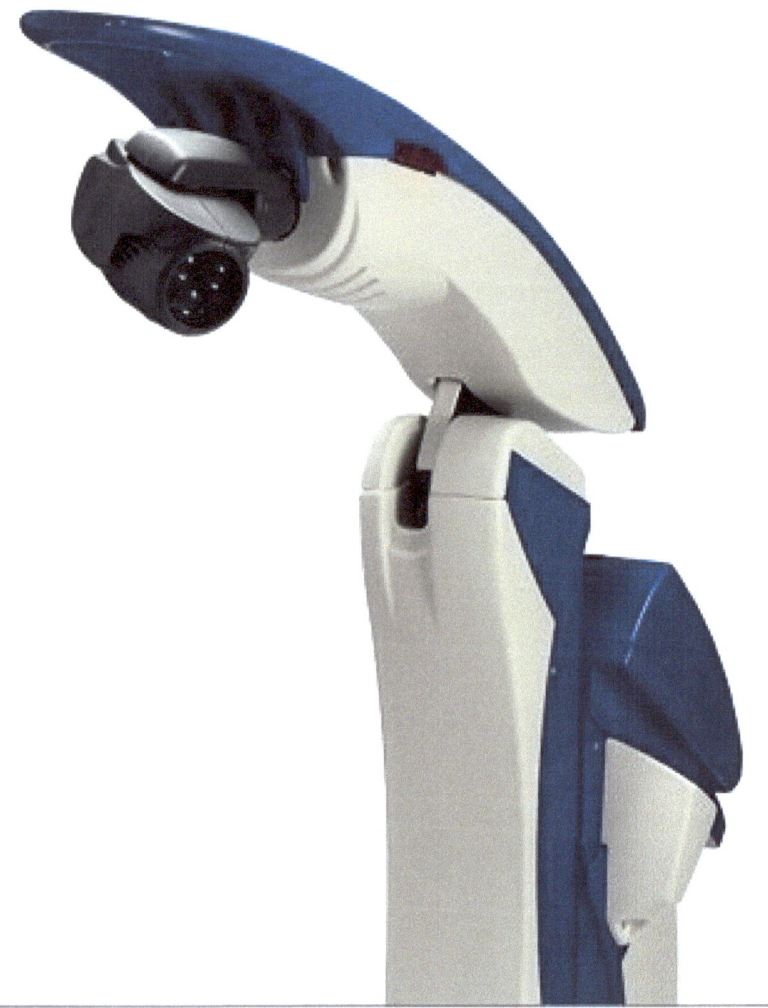

The BIORAY (biolightmedicine.com)

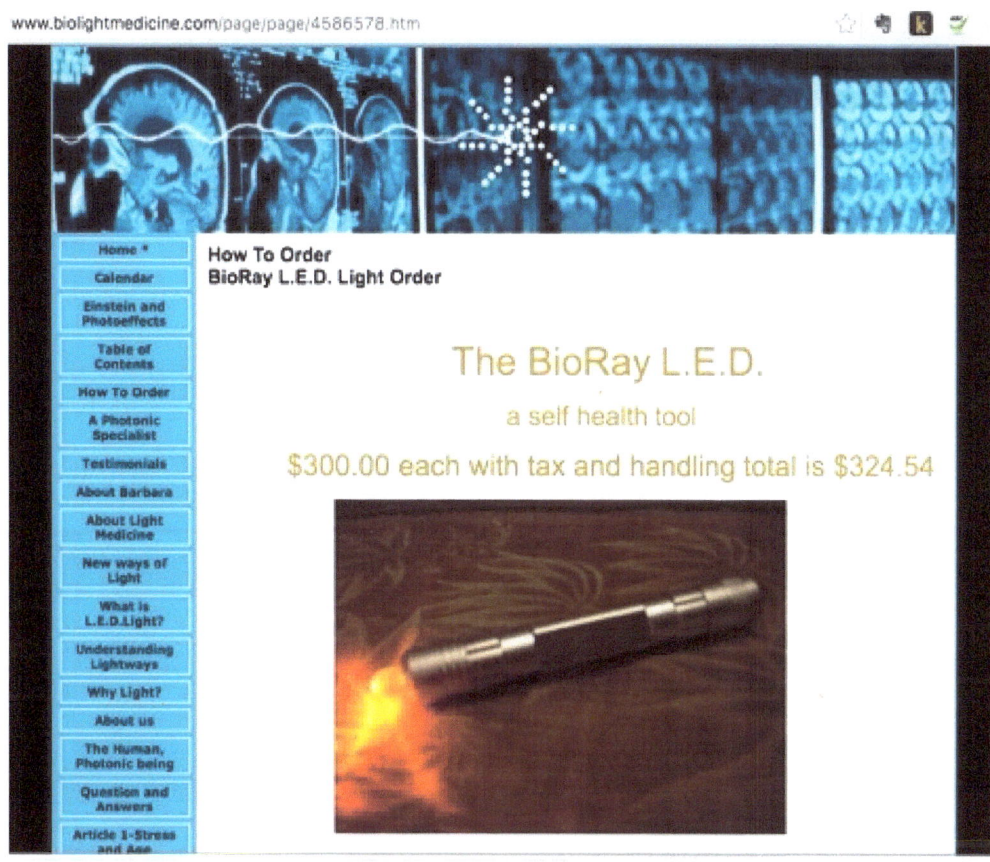

This clever design features a 660 nanometer light, battery operated and portable, which has a lens at the tip which is just the right size that you can insert it into your nose, your ear, or your naval, and energize blood and tissue. Sold by a light practitioner who uses it as an accupuncturist might, it shows that it is not necessarily the power of the device.

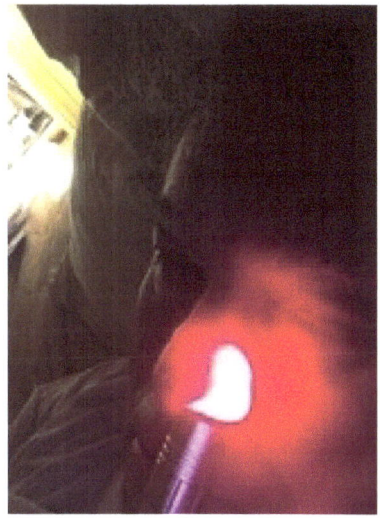

See how this device lights up much skin area when shining it into the nasal cavity.

Other devices and experiments

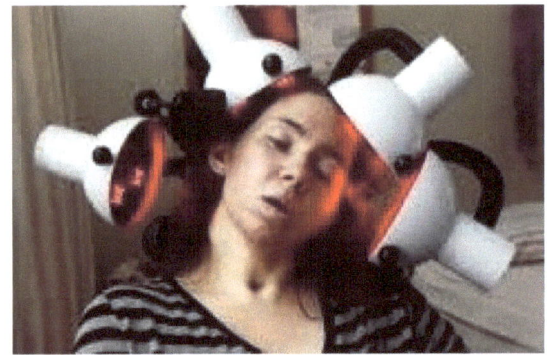

Emerson's multi-lite device

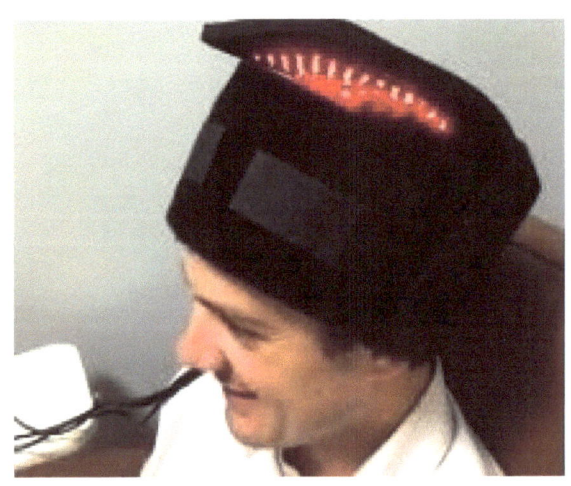

Cerescan IR trial for TBI

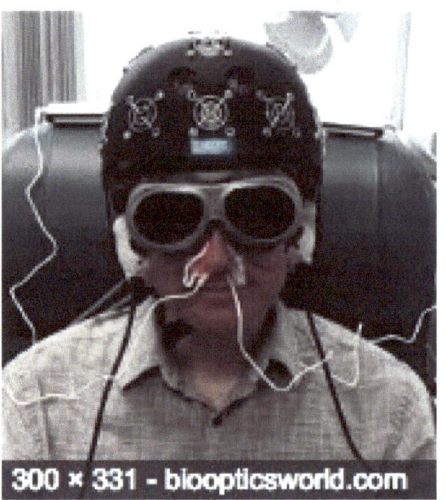

Veteran's Administration
Experimental Light Helmet,
with light in the nasal cavities,
as well. Margaret Naeser, Ph.D.

ULTRASOUND AND ALZHEIMER'S THERAPY

http://anesth.medicine.arizona.edu/tus
http://www.sciencealert.com/new-alzheimer-s-treatment-fully-restores-memory-function

Photobiomodulation is not alone in getting sufficient energy supplement to the brain. Ultrasound devices found in every hospital put out just enough energy, set to the right frequency, to help those with Alzheimer's and TBI.

Stuart Hameroff, MD, and anesthesiologist at the U of A Medical Center , has led much of the world's study of consciousness. His work on micro-tubules in neurons led to his successful experiments using low energy ultrasound imaging devices found in every hospitals to try out a therapy helping Alzheimer's patients.

I have attached information on expanded clinical trials that you can apply for. It will help explain the care and detail that these trials require, and why they need funding to move forward.

References:

Hameroff S, Trakas M, Duffield C, Annabi E, Gerace MB, Boyle P, Lucas A, Amos Q, Buadu A, Badal JJ. Transcranial ultrasound (TUS) effects on mental states: a pilot study. Brain Stimul, 2013; May; 6(3):409-15.

Sanguinetti JL, Smith E, Allen John JB, Hameroff S, (2014) Human Brain Stimulation with Transcranial Ultrasound: Potential Applications for Mental Health. Bioelectromagnetic and Subtle Energy Medicine, 2nd edition, CRC Press, pp 355-360

Leininga G, Gotz J (2015) Scanning ultrasound removes amyloid-β and restores memory in an Alzheimer's disease mouse model Science Translational Medicine 7:278-833

Bocchi L, Branca JV, Pacini S, Ruggiero M (2015) Effect of ultrasounds on neurons a nd microglia: Cell viability and automatic analysis of cell morphology, Biomedical Signal Processing and Control 22:44-53

from the University of Arizona. A study awaiting funding:

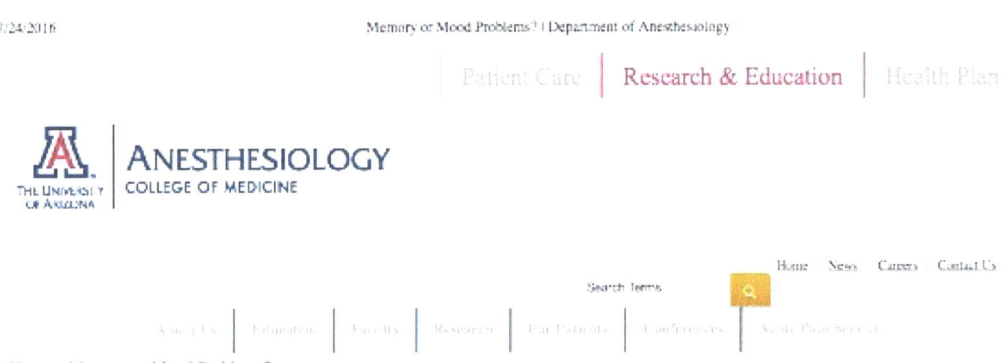

Home » Memory or Mood Problems?

Memory or Mood Problems?

Clinical Trial of Transcranial Ultrasound ('TUS')

Patients with memory, mood or cognitive problems from dementia, Alzheimer's, head injury or other brain disorders are invited to enter a free clinical trial of painless, non-invasive brain ultrasound.

Physician or self-referral

- Individuals may self-refer by contacting the Department of Anesthesiology at (520) 235-0510
- Physician may refer patients by contacting the Department at (520) 235-0510

The Department of Anesthesiology and Center for Consciousness Studies at BUMC, and the Department of Psychology at UA are sponsoring an 'open label' trial of transcranial ultrasound ('TUS') for memory, mood and cognitive disorders in patients with dementia, Alzheimer's disease and traumatic brain injury. Administered from the fronto-temporal scalp ('temporal window'), brief, low intensity TUS is safe, painless and shown to enhance mood in hundreds of human volunteers at the University of Arizona. In the lab, ultrasound increases synaptic connections, and improves symptoms and pathology in mice with genetically-induced Alzheimer's. In this study, patients will perform brief cognitive tests before and after low intensity TUS, 2 minutes per day, several days per week for several weeks.

Study Investigators

- Stuart Hameroff, MD - Anesthesiology, Banner University Medical Center - Tucson
- Jay Sanguinetti & John JB Allen, PhD - Psychology, University of Arizona
- Michael Lemole, MD - Neurosurgery, Banner University Medical Center - Tucson

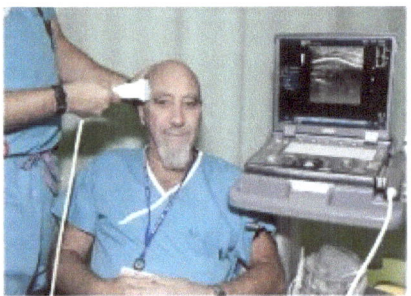

Figure 1 Transcranial Ultrasound ('TUS') from temporal window at 8 MHz with a GE diagnostic imaging device.

67

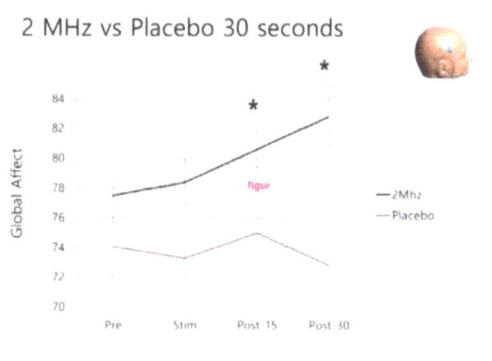

2 MHz vs Placebo 30 seconds

Global Affect

—2Mhz
—Placebo

Pre   Stim   Post-15   Post-30

Sanguinetti et al., under review

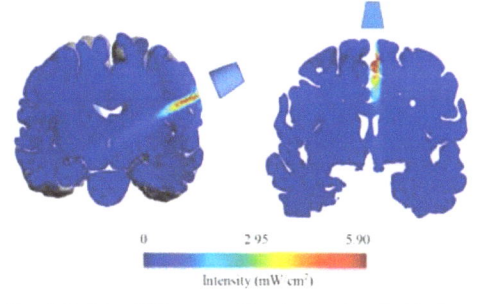

Figure 2. Simulation of TUS penetration delivered at the scalp at 150 mW cm² at temporal window (left) and vertex (right)

Intensity (mW cm²)
0   2.95   5.90

Introduction/Background

Memory and cognitive dysfunction in people with brain disorders, including Alzheimer's disease and traumatic brain injury, are enormous problems.

Various drugs, brain stimulation and training programs have been tried with minimal success. These include non-invasive transcranial direct current stimulation (tDCS, e.g. Fregni 2005), and transcranial magnetic stimulation (TMS). tDCS creates a weak electric current in the brain from electrodes placed on the scalp, and has had some success in improving verbal working memory. TMS imposes a magnetic field in the brain, and has shown promise for some cognitive symptoms of depression. But both tDCS and TMS are inconsistent, have poor spatial resolution and lack known neurophysiological mechanisms of action. A third technique is transcranial ultrasound (TUS). Ultrasound consists of mechanical vibrations, usually in low megahertz (MHz), used for many years in medical imaging. But ultrasound has also been shown to stimulate excitable nerve and muscle tissue since Harvey's studies in 1929. More recently Tyler (2011), Bystritsky (2015), Yoo (2011) and others have shown electrophysiological and behavioral effects of brain ultrasound, and our group (Hameroff et al, 2012) was the first to show effects of TUS on mental states in human volunteers. Applied at the scalp and aimed at the brain at low intensities, and for reasonably brief durations, TUS is painless and safe. TUS is significantly attenuated by the skull, with lower frequencies (e.g. 2 MHz or less) penetrating more readily. Approximately 3 percent reaches the brain to echo back through the skull for surface images (Figures 1 and 2).

Regarding safety, high intensity ultrasound can heat and cavitate tissue, and is used to cause therapeutic destructive lesions. Mid-range TUS intensities can open the blood brain barrier. On the contrary, we use low intensity, sub-thermal TUS (~150 mW/cm2) aimed at augmenting natural brain activities. The FDA has designated an ultrasound thermal threshold at 720 mW/cm2. Sub-thermal TUS (~150 mW/cm2) can safely and painlessly stimulate brain activity without long-term effects or damage (Dalecki, 2007). Simulation (Figure 2) suggests scalp levels of 150 mW/cm2 results in peak brain levels of ~6 mW/cm2.

Moreover TUS can be pulsed (on-off cycles at arbitrary frequencies and patterns), and used in either focused or unfocused beams or scanning modes. Using low intensity, sub-thermal TUS levels, we published the first study of TUS on human mood using 8 MHz TUS in a double blind protocol (Hameroff et al, 2012; Sanguinetti et al, 2014).

15 seconds of 8 MHz TUS at temporal window resulted in ~ 1 hour mood enhancement, measured by visual analog mood scale ratings, in a double blind crossover study. We have continued to show that brief (e.g. 30 seconds) low intensity TUS targeting the right frontal cortex enhanced mood (Sanguinetti et al, 2015).

Other studies (e.g. Legon et al, 2014) have shown TUS enhances cognitive function in humans, and in a recent study on mice with genetically-induced Alzheimer's disease, TUS to temporal cortex restored memory deficits and reduced amyloid plaques (Leinenga and Götz 2015)

68

TUS and Mood

Using 8 MHz TUS at 150 mW/cm2 in a double blind protocol, our group published the first study of TUS on human mood (Hameroff et al, 2012, c.f. Sanguinetti et al, 2014a; 2014b). We have continued to show that brief (e.g. 30 seconds) low intensity TUS from the scalp at the 'temporal window' aimed at right prefrontal cortex (PFC) results in approximately an hour of enhanced mood, as measured by subjective scales in randomized double blind trials (Sanguinetti et al, 2015). Other studies (e.g. Legon et al, 2014) have shown TUS enhances cognitive function in humans, and in a recent study in mice with genetically-induced Alzheimer's disease, TUS applied to temporal cortex restored memory deficits (Leinenga and Götz 2015).

With IRB approval, we have completed 3 previous clinical TUS studies on several hundred healthy human subjects without problems. The current study proposes to test effects of brief, sub-thermal TUS for memory, mood and cognition in patients with memory and/or cognitive dysfunction following brain injury (including concussion), and those who have, or may have, Alzheimer's disease or other dementia. In this experiment, patients with memory dysfunction possibly due to dementia including Alzheimer's disease and brain injury (including concussion) will be given ultrasound for cognitive enhancement and mood improvements. Studies in cell culture show brief, low intensity ultrasound accelerates neuronal growth and synaptic formation (ref). But the mechanism by which low intensity TUS affects cognitive function and mental states is unknown. Suggestions include stimulation of mechano-sensitive membrane receptors, and enhanced vibrations of cytoskeletal microtubules, known to have megahertz resonance dynamics. 2 MHz stimulation causes optimized polymerization of microtubules, which are disrupted in Alzheimer's disease and brain injury.

TUS is painless and safe when properly administered, improves mood in humans and Alzheimer's symptoms and pathology in mice. It is potentially beneficial in brain disorders, and appears to cause no harm. The time is right. As world leaders in clinical TUS, we propose to test effects of brief, sub-thermal TUS on cognitive tests for memory and mood in patients with dementia and brain injury. Although our previous studies have been double blinded, we choose here an open label approach. We recognize a possible placebo response, but also see a potential stress response, e.g. for potentially confused subjects. So we'll start with an open label 'pilot study' and consider a subsequent double blind study.

Study Protocol
Subjects with memory and cognitive dysfunction can be referred from physicians throughout Banner-University Medical Center and elsewhere. Referred subjects with a history of dementia, Alzheimer's and/or brain trauma will be pre-screened by phone. 'Alzheimer's' will be considered to include patients in any stage of Alzheimer's previously diagnosed by medical professionals at BUMC or elsewhere. Subjects with mild-to-moderate brain injury including concussion will be solicited from Neurosurgery (e.g. Dr Lemole), Neurology (e.g. Dr Hishaw), Sports Medicine and elsewhere. Overall, approximately 60 dementia and 60 head injury patients are sought.

Those with a recent history of major medical conditions (< 6 months) will be excluded. Major medical conditions include: heart attack, stroke, trauma, respiratory distress (pneumonia or other serious lung conditions), organ failure, or cancer. Patients with migraines will also be excluded.

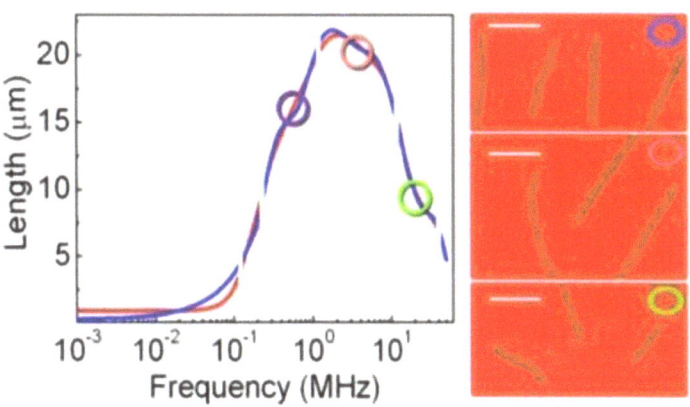

Figure 3. The mechanism of TUS is unknown, but self-assembly of microtubules, major component of neuronal cytoskeleton, is optimized at 2 MHz stimulation (Sahu et al, 2014). TUS may resonate microtubules.

The study will take place in the Center for Consciousness Studies (CCS) offices, rooms 105, 105a and 105c, in the Faculty Office Building (FOB) 1609 Warren St (directly across from the BUMC Emergency Department). FOB allows easy ground floor access and parking. Room 105 is a common area, and 105a and 105c are private rooms. The actual TUS will be conducted privately in 105a and 105c during which participants will interact only with researchers.

Upon arrival and entry to the study, subjects or their caretakers will be asked to complete intake information, written consent will be obtained, vital signs taken, and the pre-test cognitive test battery given (see below).

Patients will receive two minutes of low intensity TUS to the right and two minutes to the left temporal window twice a week for four weeks. A full battery of tests will be administered at the beginning and end of the four weeks, and a minor test battery after each exposure. Results will be assessed through pre-and post-TUS test scores, and comments from caretakers and patients.

In this study we will use a GE Logiq E imaging ultrasound (Figure 1) in broad beam scanning mode at 2 MHz, aimed roughly at pre-frontal and medial temporal cortex using sphenoid ridge as a landmark. These areas are considered key to memory in Alzheimer's disease, and executive function in brain injury.

The significance of TUS benefits would be profound, as (1) TUS is painless, safe, inexpensive, and could be widely available, and (2) memory and cognitive dysfunction in dementia and brain injury currently have no effective methods to improve cognition.

All procedures are done for research purposes. No standard care is provided to patients.

Week 1
On the first day, patients will fill out an intake form and medical intake form (see appendix 7a and 7b). Patients will be given the ADAS-Cog test while the caretakers complete the ADCS-ADL life satisfaction scale (1.6), which will take about an hour. They will also be given the cognitive tasks outlined in section 1.5 below. Patients will then receive ultrasound stimulation on the right and left temporal windows for two minutes at intensity well below the FDA limit.

On day 2 (week 1), they will be given the cognitive tasks outlined in 1.5 below. Patients will then receive ultrasound stimulation on the right and left temporal windows for two minutes.

Week 2

On days 3-4 (week 2), they will be given the cognitive tasks outlined in 1.5 below. Patients will then receive ultrasound stimulation on the right and left temporal windows for two minutes on each day.

Week 3

On days 5-6 (week 3), they will be given the cognitive tasks outlined in 1.5 below. Patients will then receive ultrasound stimulation or sham stimulation(?) on the right and left temporal lobes for two minutes.

Week 4

On days 7-8 (week 4), they will be given the cognitive tasks outlined in 1.5 and the ADAS-Cog (patients) and ADCS-ADL (caretakers) outlined in 1.6 below. Patients will then receive ultrasound stimulation or sham stimulation(?) on the right and left temporal windows for two minutes. Caretakers will repeat the ADCS-ADL at this session(repetitive?).

Cognitive and Mood Tasks

On each day, participants will perform the following simple cognitive tasks on paper or on computer:

Digit span (forward and backward) task (10-15 min): Digit span is used to assess working memory. Participants are briefly shown an increasing amount of digits and prompted to sequentially repeat the digits back to the researcher. Successful recollections will result in increasing lengths of digits until the participant is no longer successful. This can be done by repeating from the beginning to the end or then end to the beginning of the digits shown.

Trail making A and B test (5-15 min): Trail making tests the domain of executive function. In Part A, participants are given a form with scattered encircled numbers (1-25). The objective of the test is to connect the numbers in increasing order. The time taken to complete the test is measured. Part B introduces letters, alongside numbers, in the test. Participants will then connect 1 to A to 2 to B to 3 to C and so on in order to complete the test.

Word list learning (10-20 min): Word list learning is a straightforward task that tests episodic memory by asking participants to recall a list of words. The list is presented three times to the participant, each time asking the participant to repeat the words back following each word shown. After several minutes have passed the participant is asked to repeat as many words back. Recall is again tested several minutes after the first recall session. The number of correct recalls will be measured. Each day's testing will have different word lists to account for learning effects.

Paired associates learning task (10-25 min): The paired associate learning task also tests for episodic memory, associative memory. Participants are shown Two lists of words and tasked to learn the words. They are then instructed to learn randomly-paired words from the earlier task and later recall these arbitrary pairings. This is done in a manner similar to word recall.

Word recognition task (10-20 min): Similar to the free recall task, word recognition tests episodic memory. Participants are shown a list of 12 words and asked to repeat back to the researcher. Unlike the free recall task, participants will only be given one instance to learn this list. After 5 minutes participants are asked to distinguish words from a list of 24 words, 12 of which are from the initial list and 12 are new words. The number of correct responses will be measured.

Object knowledge task (5-15 min): The object knowledge task is used to test for mainly semantic memory. Participants will be shown 12 objects, four of which have frequent exposure, four with medium exposure, and four with low exposure, and asked to name the object. This is repeated for naming each finger on the hand. They can be given clues to each object's function, as specified by the ADAS-Cog manual. Participants will not be allowed to touch the objects.

Category fluency task (5-15 min): Category fluency tests for semantic memory in participants. They are given a minute to list as many words from a given category. Examples of such categories are animals, vehicles, and household items. A recording of this task will be done for future scoring purposes.

4 Mountains task (10-20 min): The 4 Mountains task is given to participants as a measure of spatial memory. A computer-generated landscape with four distinct mountains is shown to participants. Following a 2 second exposure to a blank screen, four panels are shown. One of the panels shows the initial mountain configuration, modified by reorientation and/or non-spatial features (vegetation, lighting, environment, etc.) while the other three panels will show similarly modified images of different mountains. A training phase will be given prior to actual administration. This can also be done with images printed on paper and given accordingly.

Block design task (5-15 min): Used in the Wechsler Adult Intelligence Test, the block design task measures spatial capabilities. Participants are given 16 cubes that are half red and white such that a line divides the colors at four vertices and two faces of the cube are completely red, completely white, and white and red. Participants are then given a 4x4 design and asked to replicate the design with all cubes. The amount of time taken to replicate the design is used to gauge performance.

Visual Analogue Mood Scale: A simple self-report scale. On a single sheet of paper, patients rate their current mood on six dimensions: Alertness, Sadness, Tenseness, Happiness, Weariness, Calmness, and Sleepiness. They will mark their answer along a 100mm line, from "Very Little" to "Very Much."

1.6 ADAS-Cog (60-75 min; appendix 8): The Alzheimer's Disease Assessment Scale- Cognition is a standardized cognitive battery used commonly in NIH-funded trials for Alzheimer's Disease. The domains that are tested by word recall, commands, constructional praxis, naming, ideational praxis, orientation, and word recognition. The majority of these tasks are administered in less than 5-10 minutes.

ADCS-ADL (15-20 min): The Alzheimer's Disease Cooperative Study - Activities of Daily Living measures quality of life from the caretaker's perspective. Like the ADAS-Cog, the ADL is also a standardized assessment commonly used in AD trials. The ADL consists of less than forty questions that can be administered briefly.

Since they will be aware of the study hypotheses before the experiment begins, there will be no need for a debriefing.

After one month, and again after three months, caretakers will be given a follow-up phone call and asked the questions from the ADCS-ADL.

Cost to subjects
Subjects will incur no cost during this study except their time.

Risks to subjects
Both devices (GE Logiq E, U+) are non-significant risk devices with parameters well under FDA limits for transcranial ultrasound devices (see appendix 9 for U+, and appendix 10 and 11 for manuals). The outputs for U+ were tested with a hydrophone by Russ Witte, PhD, who runs the Experimental Ultrasound and Neural Imaging Laboratory in Radiology.

The FDA limits diagnostic ultrasound to 720 mW/cm2 for adults. Above these doses, ultrasound can potentially damage tissue. Ultrasound stimulation has also been shown to be safe as studies have found effects using intensities as low as 24 W/cm2 and 150 mW/cm2, both of which are well below the 700 mW/cm2 intensity FDA allows for safe non-thermal ultrasound (i.e., the intensity used in imaging ultrasound). Thermal ultrasound refers to intensities that could damage tissue or skin.

Both ultrasound devices can only administer doses well below the approved FDA guidelines for safe human application. Therefore, it will not be possible to administer a harmful dose of the ultrasound to participants using this device.
See the 2008 FDA guidelines on ultrasound:
http://www.fda.gov/downloads/MedicalDevices/DeviceRegulationandGuidance/GuidanceDocuments/UCM070911.pdf
Both ultrasound devices emit pulsed ultrasound. The ultrasound transducer will administer a single pulse lasting for only a few seconds, repeated over two minutes. Thus the transducer will be placed on the participant's head for two minutes at a time, but the stimulation will be not continuous throughout this time. This means the actual "dose" will be minimal. We have chosen the smallest dose we expect an effect in order to minimize risk to the participants as much as possible. Ultrasound has been used in countless settings on human tissue for over 50 years and has an excellent safety record over; it has been used by the PI hundreds of times in clinical settings. We will stay far below the FDA recommended dosages and will report any unforeseen adverse outcomes immediately to the IRB. All stimulation will be 2 MHz or below at intensity well below 720 mW/cm2 which is deemed safe under the FDA guidelines and verified by published literature as a safe dose.

The ultrasound gel used on the transducer is hypoallergenic, but nonetheless could cause a very mild skin reaction in some subjects. This is very unlikely, but in the case that a researcher notices a mild reaction, or a subject complains of irritation, the study will be stopped immediately.

Potential benefits to subjects and/or society
The possible implications are wide-reaching if TUS improves memory and cognition in patients with memory and cognitive deficits in Alzheimer's, age-related decline in memory function, and brain trauma. Safe, painless and inexpensive, TUS offers potential benefit for a wide range of mental and cognitive brain disorders.

Protection of subject privacy: The entire study will take place in a private room in the Center for Consciousness Studies FOB 105. The door to the room will be shut and experimenters will ensure subject privacy. All contact via telephone or e-mail will be to schedule participants, and no identifiable or personal information will be asked in email. Therefore, should participants share an e-mail or phone line, no private information will be gleaned from our communications.

Protection of data confidentiality: Consent forms will be stored in Babcock 1114 until the end of the study. Per psychology department guidelines, at the end of the study all consent forms will be moved to the Psychology main office, room 312. Each participant will be given a unique participant identifying number that will not be recorded on his or her consent form. This unique participant number (and not any identifying information) will only be recorded on all experimental data collected. Therefore, all of the data in Babcock 1114 will be de-identified. The date of the participant's intake will be recorded on the consent form. This date will also be recorded in an Excel sheet of de-identified participant data. Consent forms will be stored in Psychology for six years should data ever need to be re-identified, as requested by the IRB. De-identified data will be secured indefinitely in electronic form on Dr. Allen's secure server. Paper copies, with no identifying information, will be shredded once entered onto the server.

Subject compensation
Patients will receive no payment for their time.

Withdrawal of subjects
Subjects will be reminded they can withdraw themselves from the study at any point if they feel uncomfortable with any part of the study design. Incomplete data will be analyzed.

Future use and long-term storage of data or specimens
As mentioned in Protection of Data Confidentiality, de-identified experimental data will be stored in a secure server belonging to Dr. John Allen. This data includes mood change, cognitive performance, quality of life, and consent forms of each subject. Physical copies will be shredded per regulation after the data is secure on Dr. Allen's server. All forms of data will not have any identifying information and will not be sold or shared with any pharmaceutical companies.

This is an 'open label', open enrollment study: All patients with memory problems attributable to dementia (including Alzheimer's) and brain injury (including concussion) – will be recruited for this study.

The caretakers of dementia patients will be recruited alongside their patient. Our rationale for an open label study is the following. For subjects with memory and cognitive impairment, visits will be both stressful and excitatory. Although the excitatory aspect of the visit could induce a placebo effect, visits are also stressful and we want to minimize untoward effects. If we see improvement we will then consider a double blind study.

An Institutional Review Board responsible for human subjects research at The University of Arizona reviewed this research project and found it to be acceptable, according to applicable state and federal regulations and University policies designed to protect the rights and welfare of participants in research.

References
Bystritsky a., Korb a. S. A Review of Low-Intensity Transcranial Focused Ultrasound for Clinical Applications. Curr Behav Neurosci Reports 2015:60–6. doi: 10.1007/s40473-015-0039-0.

Hameroff S, Trakas M, Duffield C, Annabi E, Gerace MB, Boyle P, et al. Transcranial ultrasound (TUS) effects on mental states: A pilot study. Brain Stimul 2013;6:409–15. doi:10.1016/j.brs.2012.05.002

Legon W, Sato TF, Opitz A, Mueller J, Barbour A, Williams A, et al. Transcranial focused ultrasound modulates the activity of primary somatosensory cortex in humans. Nat Neurosci 2014;17:322–9. doi:10.1038/nn.3620.

Leinenga, Gerhard, and Jürgen Götz. "Scanning ultrasound removes amyloid-β and restores memory in an Alzheimer's disease mouse model." Science translational medicine 7.278 (2015): 278ra33-278ra33.

Yoo, Seung-Schik, et al. "Focused ultrasound modulates region-specific brain activity." Neuroimage 56.3 (2011): 1267-1275.

ABOUT THE AUTHOR

Michael L. Weiner started his business career at Xerox Corporation in 1975, eventually moving the marketing headquarters in Rochester, NY, where worked in sales compensation planning, and then software marketing.

While at Xerox, Mike got license to Xerox PARC compression technology and published the Word Finder thesaurus to great market acclaim and popularity. Print rights were licensed and published by Pocket Books. The thesaurus was bundled in word processing software, and in many devices, including new handheld computers that preceded the current revolution.

Mike was an early innovator in handheld computers, and natural language processing, before joining forces with pacemaker pioneer, Wilson Greatbach*. Together they tackled the problem of making pacemakers safe instead of contraindicated for MRI, worked with industry and the FDA via a CRADA, eventually selling the technology to Medtronic for low 8 figures.

In 2010, on a trip to Vienna, Austria, Mike met with technology expert Armin Bernhard, Ph.D. an an inventor of one of the cochlear implants, who first alerted Mike that Alzheimer's and other CNS diseases appeared to do an energy deficiency, which could be resolved with non-invasive energy, delivered transcranially and non-invasively

Back in the US, Mike learned of Marvin Berman, Ph.D.'s pioneering work combining photo-biomodulation in combination with neurofeedback, for a revolutionary solution to Alzheimer's.

Mike learned of research led by Dallas Hack, MD, heading Neuroscience for the US Army, who led research in TBI that lead to the discovery that infrared light was helping soldiers with TBI. This book is to provide the community of concerned citizens, scientists, and clinicians, needed information on where a promising solution is now hiding in plain sight. Public and media awareness of this opportunity should very much help move it forward.

Mike lives in Estero, Florida, north of Naples. He can be reached at info@electrohealing.com.
bio: www.lifeboat.com/ex/bios.michael.l.weiner

https://www.linkedin.com/pulse/definitive-proof-working-solution-alzheimers-ignored-industry-weiner?trk=pulse_spock-articles

https://www.linkedin.com/in/michaelweiner

Mike's mentor (RIP):

*http://www.electrohealing.com/about/wilson-greatbatch-memorial/greatbatch-articles/

www.ingramcontent.com/pod-product-compliance
Lightning Source LLC
Chambersburg PA
CBHW050737180526
45159CB00003B/1254